HOW TO DO PRIMARY CARE EDUCATIONAL RESEARCH

WONCA Family Medicine

About the Series

The WONCA Family Medicine series is a collection of books written by world-wide experts and practitioners of family medicine, in collaboration with The World Organization of Family Doctors (WONCA).

WONCA is a not-for-profit organization and was founded in 1972 by member organizations in 18 countries. It now has 118 Member Organizations in 131 countries and territories with membership of about 500,000 family doctors and more than 90% of the world's population.

Primary Health Care around the World: Recommendations for International Policy and Development

Chris van Weel, Amanda Howe

How To Do Primary Care Research

Felicity Goodyear-Smith, Bob Mash

Every Doctor: Healthier Doctors = Healthier Patients

Leanne Rowe, Michael Kidd

Family Medicine: The Classic Papers

Michael Kidd, Iona Heath, Amanda Howe

International Perspectives on Primary Care Research

Felicity Goodyear-Smith, Bob Mash

The Contribution of Family Medicine to Improving Health Systems: A Guidebook from the World Organization of Family Doctors

Michael Kidd

How To Do Primary Care Educational Research: A Practical Guide

Mehmet Akman, Valerie Wass, Felicity Goodyear-Smith

For more information about this series, please visit: https://www.crcpress.com/WONCA-Family-Medicine/book-series/WONCA

HOW TO DO PRIMARY CARE EDUCATIONAL RESEARCH

A Practical Guide

EDITED BY

Mehmet Akman, MD, MPH, FP

Professor of Family Medicine
Department of Family Medicine
Marmara University
Istanbul, Turkey

Val Wass, OBE, MHPE, PFHEA, FAoME, PhD, FRCGP, FRCP

Professor of Medical Education in Primary Care
University of Aberdeen, Aberdeen, Scotland
Emeritus Professor of Medical Education
Faculty of Medicine and Health Sciences
University of Keele, Staffordshire, United Kingdom

Felicity Goodyear-Smith, MBChB, MD, FRNZCGP(Dist)

Department of General Practice and Primary Health Care
The University of Auckland
Auckland, New Zealand

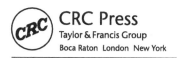

CRC Press
Taylor & Francis Group
Boca Raton London New York

CRC Press is an imprint of the
Taylor & Francis Group, an **informa** business

First edition published 2022
by CRC Press
6000 Broken Sound Parkway NW, Suite 300, Boca Raton, FL 33487-2742

and by CRC Press
2 Park Square, Milton Park, Abingdon, Oxon, OX14 4RN

© 2022 Taylor & Francis Group, LLC

CRC Press is an imprint of Taylor & Francis Group, LLC

ISBN: 9780367627102 (hbk)
ISBN: 9780367627041 (pbk)
ISBN: 9781003110460 (ebk)

Typeset in Minion Pro
by KnowledgeWorks Global Ltd.

Contents

Foreword

As a WONCA leader, one of my main commitments is to advocate for primary care, making people understand why the multidisciplinary team with a highly trained family doctor is a prerequisite to reach Universal Health Coverage.

Family medicine is a specialty in its own right, with its own curriculum and research base, and has a foundation which is different from other clinical specialties in medicine. First, we define our specialty in terms of personal relationships, in particular the patient-doctor relationship. Secondly, our diagnostic approach is defined by the patient's needs and subjective complaints, not diagnostic labels nor organ-specific diseases. These are shared values of good primary care. Continuity of care provided by the primary care team is a tool, an enzyme, which facilitates better health, and better health outcomes, in the populations we serve.

The role of the family doctor in the primary care team is first to provide value-based medical care to individuals and the community. But just as important, together with the other team members, we are educators and trainers, not only for future family doctors, but for the whole primary care team.

In our times, fragmentation, specialisation and commercialisation are dominating trends in society in general, and in health care in particular. This development challenges the core values of integrated primary care, and efforts must be made to help us stand our ground. To achieve that, training of team members must happen in the primary care setting.

To teach and train efficiently requires a certain set of contextual and value-based skills. Rapid development in technology calls for new ways of communication, in training as well as in clinical settings.

To succeed in recruiting and training health professionals in primary care, we need evidence-based methods and educational programmes. Evidence of how to teach and train, conveyed in the international language of scientific methodology, is a prerequisite to ensure that primary care disciplines are included in the curricula in postgraduate training of health care professionals.

Primary care disciplines offer a different language from the narrow specialties, and in understanding of human health. The two approaches complement one another. Because we train each other, an understanding of the principles of training in primary care should be included in postgraduate training, not only for family doctors to be, but for physicians training for all parts of the health system.

A textbook on principles of research on education in primary care disciplines is an invaluable contribution to raise awareness, and to educate and train physicians and other health care workers adequately, and help us identify success factors and failures.

This foreword is written at the end of the "First Corona Pandemic Year". We have challenges ahead, and primary care professionals will continue to take care of patients as first responders in health care. Research questions on education and training will continue to queue up in the light of the pandemic.

I am deeply grateful to the WONCA Working Parties on Research and Education for the efforts made for this book to come true. To be a primary care professional of high quality, evidence-based training is key. This book offers an easily accessible introduction to the main principles of how research can help us improve as educators and trainers.

Anna Stavdal
WONCA President Elect
Oslo, Norway

Editors

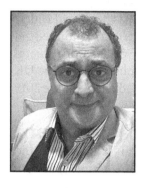

Mehmet Akman, MD, MPH, FP, is a general practitioner and professor working in the field of primary care. He has a family medicine background, received a master degree in public health, and has an extensive experience as a tutor in under- and postgraduate medical education, primary care and educational research. He is the incoming Chair of the WONCA (World Family Doctors) Working Party on Research, and a member of the Board of Trustees of the Turkish Foundation of Family Medicine (TAHEV). He was an advisory board member of the European Forum for Primary Care between 2013 and 2019 and is an associate editor of the journal *Primary Health Care Research and Development.*

Dr Akman's recent works are mainly about organisation of primary care, multi-professional primary care research, chronic disease management at the primary care level and postgraduate training of family doctors. He is involved in international research and projects as a national coordinator, advisor or research coordinator. He has served as consultant for the World Health Organization for assessment of primary care services and capacity building of health care professionals. He is the leading or co-author of more than 60 national and international articles published in peer-reviewed scientific journals, including primary care educational research, and over 10 chapters in medical books. His present position is professor of Family Medicine at Marmara University School of Medicine, Family Medicine Department, İstanbul, Turkey.

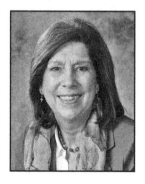

Val Wass, OBE, MHPE, PFHEA, FAoME, PhD, FRCGP, FRCP, is a general practitioner by trade. She has progressively combined clinical work with academic research throughout her UK career. Past roles include Academic Primary Care at Guy's, Kings and St Thomas' Medical School (1995–2003), Professor of Community Based Medical, University of Manchester (2003–2009) and Head of the School of Medicine at Keele University (2009–2015). She retired in 2015, to take up UK consultancy roles as

Professor of Medical Education in Primary Care at Aberdeen University and Emeritus Professor of Medical Education, Keele University. She chairs the WONCA Working Party on Education and is Chief Editor of the journal *Education for Primary Care*.

The International Masters in Health Profession Education (MHPE) and PhD at Maastricht University offered a strong platform for medical education research both undergraduate and postgraduate and she has published widely with >5,000 citations. Awards for an outstanding contribution to medical education include the United Kingdom (UK) Royal College of General Practitioners William Pickles and President's International Medals, the UK Association for the Study of Medical Education Gold Medal and, in the 2015 UK New Year's Honours, an OBE.

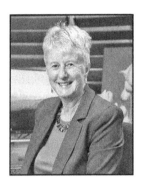 **Felicity Goodyear-Smith, MBChB, MD, FRNZCGP(Dist)** is a General Practitioner and Professor of General Practice and Primary Health Care at The University of Auckland, Auckland, New Zealand. In collaboration with Prof Bob Mash, she co-edited the two companion books to this current title: *International Perspectives in Primary Care Research* (CRC Press, 2016) and *How To Do Primary Care Research* (CRC Press, 2019). She is Chair of the WONCA Working Party on Research, and all three of these books have been written on behalf of WONCA. Dr Goodyear-Smith was the founding editor-in-chief of the *Journal of Primary Health Care*. As well as a number of books and book chapters, she has published over 270 peer-reviewed papers, including 18 on various aspects of primary care educational research.

She is passionate about the importance of research underpinning teaching and learning in primary care, to provide a solid evidence base for our educational interventions and innovations. Educational research can also serve to build the research skills of early career academics, who may have been employed to teach, but who have few research skills, enabling clinical teachers to upskill in research methodology, and be co-authors of peer-reviewed publications.

Contributors

Mehmet Akman, MD, MPH, FP
Professor
Department of Family Medicine
Marmara University
Istanbul, Turkey

Chaisiri Angkurawaranon, MD, MSc, PhD
Lecturer
Department of Family Medicine
Faculty of Medicine
Chiang Mai University
Chiang Mai, Thailand

Douglas Archibald, PhD
Associate Professor
Department of Family Medicine
University of Ottawa
Ottawa, Canada

Tracie A. Barnett, PhD
Associate Professor
Department of Family Medicine
McGill University
Montreal, Quebec, Canada

Gillian Bartlett, PhD
Professor
Department of Family and
Community Medicine
University of Missouri
Columbia, Missouri

Raquel Gómez Bravo, MD
Doctoral Researcher
Department of Behavioural and
Cognitive Sciences
University of Luxembourg
Luxembourg City, Luxembourg

Saliha Serap Cifcili, MD
Professor
Department of Family Medicine
Marmara University Medical
School
İstanbul, Turkey

Vincent K. Cubaka, MD, MMED, PhD
Director
Department of Research and
Training
Partners in Health
Rwanda

Tim Dare, PhD, MJur, LLB
Professor
Department of Philosophy
The University of Auckland
Auckland, New Zealand

Jan De Maeseneer, MD, PhD
Emeritus Professor
Department of Public Health and
Primary Care
Ghent University
Ghent, Belgium

Jamie DeMore, MA
PhD Candidate
Department of Family Medicine
McGill University
Montreal, Quebec, Canada

Jon Dowell, BMBS, DCH, DRCOG, MRCGP, MD, FHEA
Professor of General Practice
  University of Dundee
  Dundee, Scotland

Claire Duddy, BA, MA, AFHEA
Realist Reviewer
  Nuffield Department of Primary
    Care Health Sciences
  University of Oxford
  Oxford, United Kingdom

Kyle Eggleton, MBChB, MMedSci, MPH, PhD, FRNZCGP(Dist)
Rural Director
  Department of General Practice
    and Primary Health Care
  The University of Auckland
  Auckland, New Zealand

Hélène Elidor, MD, MPH, MSc
ULaval Practice Based Research
    Network (ULaval PBRN)
    Coordinator
  Department of Family Medicine
  Université Laval
  Quebec, Canada

John Epling, MD, MSEd
Professor
  Department of Family and
    Community Medicine
  Virginia Tech Carilion School of
    Medicine
  Roanoke, Virginia

Michael D. Fetters, MD, MPH, MA
Director
  Mixed Methods Program and
    Professor
  Department of Family Medicine
  University of Michigan
  Ann Arbor, Michigan

Simon Forrest, PhD, MA(ed), PGCE, PGCAP, BA
Professor of Sociology & Principal of
  the College of St Hild & St Bede
  Durham University
  Durham, United Kingdom

Simon Gay, MBBS, MSc, MMedEd, FRCGP, SFHEA
Professor of Medical Education
  (Primary Care)
  School of Medicine
  University of Leister
  Leister, United Kingdom

Felicity Goodyear-Smith, MBChB, MD, FRNZCGP(Dist)
Professor
  Department of General Practice
    and Primary Health Care
  The University of Auckland
  Auckland, New Zealand

Alex Harding, MEd, DEd, FRCGP
Associate Professor
  Department of Primary Care
    Research (APEX)
  University of Exeter
  Exeter, United Kingdom

Jo Hart, BSc, MSc, PhD, CPsychol PFHEA
Professor
  Division of Medical Education
  University of Manchester
  Manchester, United Kingdom

Kathryn Hoffmann, MPH
Associate Professor
  Department of Social and
    Preventive Medicine
  Center for Public Health
  Medical University of Vienna
  Vienna, Austria

Wichuda Jiraporncharoen, MD, MSc
Associate Professor
Department of Family Medicine
Faculty of Medicine
Chiang Mai University
Chiang Mai, Thailand

Jenny Johnston, PhD MRCGP
Reader
Centre for Medical Education
Queen's University Belfast
Belfast, Northern Ireland

Euan Lawson, FRCGP
Editor BJGP
Royal College of General
Practitioners
London, United Kingdom

Charilaos Lygidakis, MD, PhD
Visiting Researcher
Department of Behavioural and
Cognitive Sciences
University of Luxembourg
Luxemberg City, Luxemberg

Bob Mash, MBChB, DRCOG, DCH, FRCGP, FCFP(SA), PhD
Distinguished Professor
Division of Family Medicine and
Primary Care
Stellenbosch University
Cape Town, South Africa

Robin Miller, BSc, MSW, MSc, PhD
Professor
School of Social Policy
University of Birmingham
Birmingham, United Kingdom

Hilary Neve, MBChB, Med in Primary Health Care, MRCGP
Professor of Medical Education
Peninsula Medical School
University of Plymouth
Plymouth, United Kingdom

Sophie Park, MBChB, MMedSci(dist), SFHEA, EdD, FRCGP
Professor
Research Department of Primary
Care and Population Health
University College London
London, United Kingdom

David Ponka, MD CM, CCFP(EM), MSc, FCFP
Director
The Besrour Centre for Global
Family Medicine
The College of Family Physicians
of Canada and Associate
Professor
Department of Family Medicine
University of Ottawa
Ottawa, Canada

Peter Pype, MD, PhD
Professor
Department of Public Health and
Primary Care
Research Unit Interprofessional
Collaboration in Education and
Practice
Ghent University
Ghent, Belgium

Vivian R. Ramsden, RN, BSN, MS, PhD, MCFP(Hon)
Professor
Department of Academic Family
Medicine
University of Saskatchewan
Saskatoon, Canada

Rebecca Rees, BA(Hons), MSc, DPhil, FHEA
Associate Professor
  EPPI-Centre
  UCL Social Research Institute
  University College London
  London, United Kingdom

Helen Reid, BMBCh, BA, MA, MPhil, PhD, MRCGP
Centre for Medical Education
  Queen's University Belfast
  Belfast, Northern Ireland

Charo Rodríguez, MD, MSc, PhD
Professor
  Department of Family Medicine,
  and Associate Member
  Institute of Health Sciences
  Education
  McGill University
  Montreal, Quebec, Canada

John Sandars, MBChB(Hons), MD, MSc, MRCP, MRCGP, FAcadMEd
Professor of Medical Education
  Edge Hill University Medical
  School
  Ormskirk, United Kingdom

Katrina F. Sawchuk, BA, BEd, Med
Principal of St Mark Community
  School
Saskatoon and PhD Candidate
  Health Sciences Program
  College of Medicine
  University of Saskatchewan
  Saskatoon, Canada

Nynke Scherpbier-de Haan, MD, PhD
Associate Professor
  Department of Primary and
  Community Care
  Radboud University Medical
  Centre
  Nijmegen, the Netherlands

Maham Stanyon, MBBS, MRCGP, MRCP, DRCOG, FHEA, PGDip(Ed)
Assistant Professor
  Centre for Medical Education
  and Career Development
  Department of Community and
  Family Medicine
  Fukushima Medical University
  Fukushima, Japan

Roger Strasser, AM, MBBS, MClSc, FRACGP, FACRRM
Professor of Rural Health
  Te Huataki Waiora School of
  Health
  University of Waikato
  Hamilton, New Zealand
Professor of Rural Health
Founding Dean Emeritus
  Northern Ontario School of
  Medicine
  Lakehead and Laurentian
  Universities
  Thunder Bay and Sudbury,
  Ontario, Canada

Arzu Uzuner, MD, PhD
Professor
  Department of Family Medicine
  Marmara University
  Istanbul, Turkey

Val Wass, OBE, MHPE, PFHEA, FAoME, PhD, FRCGP, FRCP
Professor of Medical Education in Primary Care
University of Aberdeen
Aberdeen, Scotland
Emeritus Professor of Medical Education
  Faculty of Medicine and Health Sciences
  University of Keele
  Staffordshire, United Kingdom

John Yaphe, MD, MClSc
Associate Professor
  School of Medicine
  University of Minho
  Braga, Portugal

CHAPTER 1

Introduction

Felicity Goodyear-Smith,
Mehmet Akman and
Val Wass

This book aims to engage, upskill and support those interested in researching and evaluating teaching and training in primary care in both undergraduate and postgraduate settings around the world. This includes academics at various universities and institutions teaching and evaluating their own primary care programmes, as well as students, trainees and clinicians who might conduct primary care educational research for an honours dissertation or master's thesis. This will help grow academics in this discipline in high, as well as in middle- and low-income countries.

Primary care is a rapidly growing academic branch of learning, and developing its own body of research is the hallmark of a maturing academic discipline.[1] Research informs clinical practice, organisation of primary care services and also teaching the discipline. Educational practices and modes of delivery are rapidly changing, particularly in response to new information technologies. Primary care practitioners must engage in life-long learning. Teaching and learning of undergraduate medical and other health professionals, their respective vocational training and their continuing professional development, all need a robust evidence base to inform best practice.

The book explains the unique and specific nature of primary care educational research, and discusses its ontological, epistemological and methodological underpinnings. It explores the scope of primary care educational research, and the current research environment in the contexts of undergraduate education, postgraduate training, continuing professional development and patient education. It is primarily a practical 'how to' on designing, conducting and disseminating primary care educational research, especially for new and emerging researchers. It provides a step-by-step guide into the processes of literature review (establishing the existing knowledge base), choosing a topic, research question and methodology, conducting the research and disseminating it. Specific methods are clearly explained, and the book also covers building research capacity through mentoring, developing critical mass and inter-cultural collaborations.

In line with current primary care models of care involving interdisciplinary teams, there is a focus on interprofessional education. There is growing use of co-design in primary care research, to ensure that the new knowledge created meets the needs of the clinician and patient end-users.[2] Similarly, co-design of primary care educational research, and the use of participatory research approaches, can ensure that co-created knowledge is acted upon by the stakeholders – the teachers and the learners.

Conducting educational research in primary care has a number of benefits. Primarily, it provides a solid evidence base for educational interventions and innovations. Clinical academic staff, who advance the knowledge base of their discipline by conducting research and generating evidence, need to similarly apply these scientific principles to teaching and learning. Teaching and learning need to be grounded in theory and informed by evidence. It is also increasingly important to raise the standards of evaluating primary care education to investigate the impact on learning, behaviour change and, even more challenging, patient outcomes. This requires careful planning.[3]

In our discipline, evidence-based practice requires the synthesis of the best scientific evidence, our professional judgement and contextual evidence relating to our patients' unique values and circumstances.[4,5] Best clinical practice needs to be applied in the context of the individual patient. So too, best educational practice needs to take into account the context of the individual learner.

According to Van Der Vleuten et al., traditional education fails to put into practice what is known about effective learning.[6] For example, current evidence indicates that learning is not just knowledge transfer from teacher to student, it is a process that includes interaction with the environment. Just as in patient-centred care, learners are at the centre of the educational process, constructing new knowledge based on their own prior experiences and understanding. Learners have a goal when they are in a learning environment, as to why they are in a programme, or undertaking an activity. This will be a primary factor in determining what each attends to, what prior experiences they bring to bear in constructing meaning and understanding and hence what they learn.[7] The learning and application environments should be as close as possible.

There is a growing literature in medical education suggesting that reflection improves learning and performance in essential competencies. Specifically, reflective learning can improve professionalism and clinical reasoning, and reflective practice can contribute to continuous practice improvement and better management of complex health systems and patients.[8,9] Educational research may point the way towards more effective modes of delivery, or ensure that our assessments are meaningful, and aligned with our key objectives, course content and learning outcomes. It may also help us gain a better understanding of the conceptual frameworks underlying critical reflection, which will not only enable greater learning from the experience being reflected upon but develop reflective skills for life-long learning.[10]

Educational research is a valuable means to build the research skills of early career academics, who may have been employed to teach, but who have few research skills. If mentored by a more senior academic member, this can foster collective research and evaluation projects. In this way, everyone can upskill in research methodology, and be co-authors of peer-reviewed publications. Engaging the curiosity of young students and trainees in researching and evaluating their primary care teaching can prove a most effective way of building their curiosity in a future career in academic primary care. Often educational research requires little or no specific funding and can be conducted within a department's existing budget, which is another strong advantage for engaging in this type of research.

Research initiatives can range from the development of a curriculum at all levels (formal, informal and hidden); determining learning outcomes; developing appropriate assessments and feedback and evaluating the effectiveness of a programme. The feasibility, acceptability and effectiveness of different modes of course delivery, from face-to-face to asynchronous online, can be assessed. A teacher may assess the inter-rater reliability of different markers to get consistent student grading,[11] or measure how well a course meets its specified learning outcomes, and changes behaviour and clinical practice. The educational programme may be an undergraduate training curriculum in medicine, nursing or a number of other allied health professions, including community pharmacy, physiotherapy and occupational health. Aiding the researcher to understand the range of research methods and how they can be selected and enacted to investigate the complexity of interaction within a curriculum is one of our prime aims.

Methods need to match the research question. A randomised controlled trial may be used to assess the effectiveness of two different modes of delivering a programme.[12] Statistical analyses of quantitative data are appropriate to develop and assess the reliability and validity of an educational tool.[13] Content analysis of qualitative data may help determine ways to improve the learning and teaching experience of medical students.[14] Because the values and experiences of learners, as well as research evidence, are important in best educational practice, primary care educational research can lend itself to a mixed methods approach.[15] Qualitative research can add a narrative to our numbers, and the why and how to our results. This knowledge may help us understand specific contexts or relationships, and hence add meaning.[16]

Hence today a team approach in primary care has proven benefits in achieving better outcomes in many respects. Forty-five authors from different professions and countries contributed to this book in order to elaborate all the issues mentioned above, and even more. We hope this book will inspire you to undertake research in your own learning environments, and provide you with the tools to do so.

REFERENCES

1. Goodyear-Smith F. What makes research primary care research. In: Goodyear-Smith F, Mash R, eds. *How To Do Primary Care Research*. London, UK: CRC Press, Taylor & Francis Group; 2018: 3–6.
2. Goodyear-Smith F. Collective enquiry and reflective action in research: towards a clarification of the terminology. *Fam Pract* 2017;34(3):268–271.
3. Sandars J, Brown J, Walsh K. Producing useful evaluations in medical education. *Educ Prim Care* 2017;28(3):137–140.
4. Goodyear-Smith F. Practising alchemy: the transmutation of evidence into best health care. *Fam Pract* 2011;28(2):123–127.
5. Straus S, Glaziou P, Richardson S, Hayne B. *Evidence-Based Medicine E-Book: How to Practice and Teach EBM*. 5th ed. Edinburgh: Elsevier; 2019.
6. Van Der Vleuten P, Dolman D, Scherpbier A. The need for evidence in education. *Med Teach* 2000;22(3):246–250.
7. Savery JR, Duffy T. Problem based learning: an instructional model and its constructivist framework. *Educ Tech* 1995;35:31–38.
8. Mann K, Gordon J, MacLeod A. Reflection and reflective practice in health professions education: a systematic review. *Adv Health Sci Edu Theory Pract* 2009;14(4):595–621.
9. Sandars J. The use of reflection in medical education: AMEE Guide No. 44. *Med Teach* 2009;31(8):685–695.
10. Aronson L. Twelve tips for teaching reflection at all levels of medical education. *Med Teach* 2011;33(3):200–205.
11. Eggleton K, Goodyear-Smith F, Paton L, et al. Reliability of mini-CEX assessment of medical students in general practice clinical attachments. *Fam Med* 2016;48(8):624–630.
12. Elley CR, Clinick T, Wong C, et al. Effectiveness of simulated clinical teaching in general practice: randomised controlled trial. *J Prim Health Care* 2012;4(4):281–287.
13. Eggleton K, Goodyear-Smith F, Henning M, Jones R, Shulruf B. A psychometric evaluation of the University of Auckland General Practice Report of Educational Environment: UAGREE. *Med Educ* 2017;28(2):86–93.
14. Eggleton K, Fortier R, Fishman T, Hawken SJ, Goodyear-Smith F. Legitimate participation of medical students in community attachments. *Educ Prim Care* 2019;30(1):35–40.
15. Cresswell J, Plano Clark V, Guttman M, Hanson W. *Handbook on Mixed Methods in the Behavioral and Social Sciences*. Thousand Oaks, CA: Sage Publications; 2003.
16. Shannon-Baker P. Making paradigms meaningful in mixed methods research. *J Mix Method Res* 2016;10(4):319–334.

CHAPTER 2

The theoretical underpinnings of primary care educational research

Peter Pype,
Robin Miller and
Nynke Scherpbier

I suppose it is tempting, if the only tool you have is a hammer, to treat everything as if it were a nail.[1]

INTRODUCTION

Consciously or unconsciously, we all use frameworks to understand the world. These frameworks determine what we see (and what we do not see), what we view as important, how we interpret our experience and observations and our practical and intellectual responses. Often misunderstandings occur between people when we fail to acknowledge or explicitly communicate the frameworks we are using as a lens to observe and understand the world. This includes our ontological (assumptions about the nature of reality) and epistemological (assumptions about the nature of knowledge) stance. For example, positivism assumes there is one reality that can be known, and research is able to find out the true state of that reality. On the other hand, interpretivism assumes there are multiple realities, as the meaning of what we see stems from our experience and as a consequence can be multiple.

The frameworks that we adhere to and our connected worldviews guide us to theories, study designs and methods for analysis within our research programmes. Being aware of and acknowledging these worldviews becomes even more important when we are in a position with high responsibility.

People engaged with the design and delivery of education, or conducting educational research, carry such responsibility.[2] Because evidence should inform practice, both researchers and educationalists need to be aware of and communicate the theoretical frameworks they use in order to reach an effective cross-fertilisation. This will allow for theory-building to occur and to reach the ultimate purpose of primary care educational research, namely, improved health care quality and patient outcomes.[3]

THEORY IN EDUCATIONAL RESEARCH

Using theories to understand the problem, formulating a research question, and analysing or interpreting the results, allows researchers to advance the field by adding insights to existing theories.[4] A theory has been defined as *'an organized, coherent, and systematic articulation of a set of issues that are communicated as a meaningful whole'* providing *'a complex and comprehensive conceptual understanding of how things work'.*[5]

Theories have been classified in groups according to the lens they provide: humanistic (focus on the individual, e.g. reflective learning), sociocultural (focus on social and cultural context, e.g. communities of practice) and cognitive-behavioural (focus on the individual's processes of thinking, emotion and behaviour, e.g. theory of planned behaviour) that supports researchers in selecting a theory fit for purpose.[6] Hodges et al. group theories according to the disciplines they originate from: bioscience theories (e.g. cognitive load theory), learning theories (e.g. adult learning theory) and sociocultural theories (e.g. critical theories).[7] Another way of clustering theories is according to the curriculum components theories may underpin: planning, management and governance (e.g. complexity theory); faculty development (e.g. contact hypothesis and adult learning theory); learning outcomes (e.g. self-efficacy); learning activity (e.g. transformational learning); assessment (e.g. idea dominance) and evaluation (e.g. critical discourse).[8] Every way of grouping theories has its own rationale, and serves as a guidance for researchers to select a theory that can help identify the basic concepts involved in the concrete problem to be researched, and the underlying mechanisms of teaching and learning relevant to the educational problem at stake.[9] Hundreds of theories exist and often a combination of them offers the best way to frame the research project.

HEALTH EDUCATIONAL RESEARCH

Medical education is organised along a lifelong learning continuum of undergraduate learning, postgraduate training and continuing professional development to reach the ultimate goal of high-quality patient care through the delivery and support of competent health care providers. The successive educational units building the lifelong learning programme need to be informed by theories on the understanding of teaching (the science of instruction) and learning (the science of learning) gained from educational research.[10] Therefore, we need theory-based, programmatic research in which consecutive research projects are executed in coherence, rather than isolated, disjointed research projects.[11] An iterative process framed within the lifelong educational framework advances our understanding of teaching and learning while building on and adding to explicit theories.

Advancing the science of educational practice through the scientific cycle means that every step of the cycle should be subject to research. Cook et al. propose a framework for classifying the purposes of research in medical education mirroring the scientific cycle.[12] They describe three types of studies, each with their own purpose and their own method. Description studies focus on observation, the first step in the cycle. These studies describe new models, new educational interventions or new assessment methods. Justification studies focus on testing a hypothesis, the last step in the cycle, for instance comparing the efficiency of two educational interventions. Clarification studies focus on every step, building on previous research, making predictions and testing these in a qualitative way.[12] Clarification studies answer the question 'why and how does it work?' and advance our understanding through refining existing theories or conceptual models. Although all three study types are needed, there is a shortage of clarification studies in the literature and these are the ones we need to advance the field.[12] The Association for Medical Education (AMEE) describes four study types: justification, observational, explorative and translational studies.[9] Every type has its own design, reflecting its conceptual framework, worldview and purpose.

Four major research paradigms can be identified, each with their own methodologies and methods: positivism, post-positivism, interpretivism and critical theory.[13] Within these, many theories exist. The importance of the theories and conceptual frameworks underpinning educational research is stressed by the need for alignment between worldview and methodology.[9,14] In general, quantitative research stems from the positivism/post-positivism paradigm, while qualitative research originates within the constructivism/interpretivism paradigm.[15] Both have their own purpose and their own approach. Quantitative methods aim at hypothesis-testing and produce generalisable data with predictive value (see Chapter 16), while qualitative methods are more exploratory and hypothesis-generative in nature, aiming at a deeper understanding of phenomena (Chapter 20).[15] Data collection and analysis methods vary accordingly. Pragmatic use of both paradigms in the same research programme (mixed methods research [Chapter 26]) is a flexible way of triangulating data to gain deeper insight in the phenomena under research.

Guidance for reporting on training interventions in health care states that an explicit criterion is 'Description of the underlying theoretical framework'.[16] Laksov et al.[17] identified three ways of how researchers in medical education can report on the connection of their research with theory: as a close-up exploration aiming at explaining a specific phenomenon; as a specific perspective, often adding to theory-building using theoretical perspectives from fields other than health care education such as psychology or anthropology and as an overview or distant perspective, often reporting on previous research findings in a literature review. A literature review is a distinct research method with realist reviews playing an important role as they seek to answer to the question 'what works, for whom, why, and in what circumstances?'.[18]

BOX 2.1 USING THEORY TO DEVELOP AND EVALUATE IMPLEMENTATION INTERVENTIONS IN PRIMARY CARE[19]

A theory-based intervention modelling process was used to develop and evaluate an intervention to change general practices' (GPs) intentions to manage upper respiratory tract infections without prescribing antibiotics. Three psychological theories of behaviour change were selected providing theoretical constructs (e.g. beliefs) as antecedents of behaviour. These constructs were targeted by the intervention to promote the uptake of evidence-based practice. As such, the theories identify predictors of behaviour and provide measurable endpoints. Explanatory process measures were equally drawn from the same theories. The design was a randomised 2×2 factorial randomised controlled trial with baseline and post-intervention assessment. The analysis of the results offers an understanding of how and why the interventions work on changing behaviour. A clear table of theoretical constructs with matching operationalised measures is presented in the paper.

BOX 2.2 USING THEORY TO CREATE AN UNDERGRADUATE PRIMARY CARE VIRTUAL PATIENT MODEL[20]

With the theories of adult learning and self-directed learning as a background, this study aimed to create a virtual patient model to enhance students' clinical reasoning, communication skills and reflection. The model was created as a formative learning activity of iterated learning cycles containing simulated experiences based upon video material followed by a student reaction, feedback from the teacher and student reflection. The student's reflection drove the case forward. Analysis of the prototype confirmed that the model supported self-directed learning and stimulated reflection. Authors explain how students' experiences with the model fit in the theories used to design the model.

MOVING FORWARD PRIMARY CARE EDUCATIONAL RESEARCH

The systematic use and thorough reporting of theoretical and educational frameworks in primary care educational research will create a transparent overview of where we stand and identify areas where more research is needed. We will be able, for instance, to adjust the focus towards a better understanding of the nature of interprofessional collaboration and education in primary care settings, develop and assess educational interventions to prepare professionals for future health care challenges or define under-researched parts of the lifelong learning trajectory, such as interprofessional continuing development interventions. Detecting gaps in this way may inform the research agenda of the international primary care educational community. This research agenda should be a balanced masterplan containing priority topics, reflecting the entire scientific cycle and justify the choices by framing them into theoretical and educational frameworks. If the research community collectively adheres to this masterplan, we will be able to advance our field forward effectively.

FURTHER READINGS

Haig A, Dozier M. BEME Guide No 3: systematic searching for evidence in medical education–Part 1: sources of information. *Med Teach* 2003;25(4):352–363. doi:10.1080/0142159031000136815

Haig A, Dozier M. BEME Guide No. 3: systematic searching for evidence in medical education–Part 2: constructing searches. *Med Teach* 2003;25(5):463–484. doi:10.1080/0142159031000 01608667

REFERENCES

1. Maslow AH. *The Psychology of Science: A Reconnaissance.* New York: Harper & Row; 1966.
2. McMillan W. Theory in healthcare education research: the importance of worldview. In: Cleland J, Durning SJ, eds. *Researching Medical Education.* 1st ed. John Wiley & Sons; 2015: 15–23.
3. McGahie WC. Medical education research as translational science. *Sci Transl Med* 2010;2(19):19cm8. doi:10.1126/scitranslmed.3000679.
4. Rees CE, Monrouxe LV. Theory in medical education research: how do we get there? *Med Educ* 2010;44:334–339.
5. Reeves S, Albert M, Kuper A, Hodges BD. Why use theories in qualitative research. *BMJ* 2008;337(7670):631–634.
6. Brown J, Bearman M, Kirby C, Molloy E, Colville D, Nestel D. Theory, a lost character? As presented in general practice education research papers. *Med Educ* 2019;53:443–457.
7. Hodges BD, Kuper A. Theory and practice in the design and conduct of graduate medical education. *Acad Med* 2012;87: 25–33.
8. Hean S, Green C, Anderson E, Morris D, John C, Pitt R, O'Halloran C. The contribution of theory to the design, delivery and evaluation of interprofessional curricula: BEME Guide 49. *Med Teach* 2018;40: 542–558.

9. Ringsted C, Hodges B, Scherpbier A. 'The research compass': an introduction to research in medical education: AMEE Guide No. 56. *Med Teach* 2011;33:695–709.

10. Mayer RE. Applying the science of learning to medical education. *Med Educ* 2010;44:543–549.

11. Bordage G. Moving the field forward: going beyond quantitative-qualitative. *Acad Med* 2007;82:S126–S128.

12. Cook DA, Bordage G, Schmidt HG. Description, justification and clarification: a framework for classifying the purposes of research in medical education. *Med Educ* 2008;42:128–133.

13. Bunniss S, Kelly DR. Research paradigms in medical education research. *Med Educ* 2010;44:358–366.

14. Boet S, Sharma S, Goldman J, Reeves S. Review article: medical education research: an overview of methods. *Can J Anaesth* 2012;59(2):159–170.

15. Cleland J. Exploring versus measuring: considering the fundamental differences between qualitative and quantitative research. In: Cleland J, Durning SJ, eds. *Researching Medical Education*. 1st ed. John Wiley & Sons; 2015: 3–14.

16. Van Hecke A, Duprez V, Pype P, Beeckman D, Verhaeghe S. Criteria for describing and evaluating training interventions in healthcare professions – Cre-DEPTH. *Nurs Educ Today* 2020.

17. Bolander Laksov K, Dornan T, Teunissen PW. Making theory explicit – an analysis of how medical education research(ers) describe how they connect to theory. *BMC Med Educ* 2017;17:18. doi:10.1186/s12909-016-0848-1

18. Mertens F, de Groot E, Meijer L, Wens J, Gemma Cherry M, Deveugele M, Damoiseaux R, Stes A, Pype P. Workplace learning through collaboration in primary healthcare: a BEME realist review of what works, for whom and in what circumstances: BEME Guide. 46. *Med Teach* 2018;40(2):117–134.

19. Hrisos S, Eccles M, Johnston M, Francis J, Kaner EFS, Steen N, Grimshaw J. An intervention modelling experiment to change GPs' intentions to implement evidence-based practice: using theory-based interventions to promote GP management of upper respiratory tract infection without prescribing antibiotics. *BMC Health Serv Res* 2008;8:10.

20. Tran C, Toth-Pal E, Ekblad S, Fors U, Salminen H A virtual patient model for students' interprofessional learning in primary healthcare. *PLOS ONE* 2020. 15(9): e0238797

Underpinning medical education research with the disciplines of sociology and psychology

Jo Hart and Simon Forrest

This chapter explains the underpinning disciplines of sociology and psychology, and how understanding these might help you when you are developing your own research project.

WHAT IS SOCIOLOGY?

Sociology is the science of understanding society, concerned with the relationships between people, social structures and institutions and wider culture. This is sometimes thought of a mindset or as a 'way of seeing', and hence understanding the world in which we live.[1] Most sociological training is about acquiring ideas, theories and use of research methods that examine these links in various ways. The sociological 'way of seeing' which links individual experience to social factors can be very apparent – for example, in relation to how we think about the social basis, context and determinants of health.[2] The relationship between social and health inequalities illustrates how a sociological mindset and associated research methods can demonstrate the impact of privation and deprivation on health outcomes including mortality and morbidity.[3]

One of the strongest relationships between sociology and medical education comes about through the deployment of research methods widely used, and in some cases, developed within sociology. Understanding the links between these methods, the nature of the enquiry, and its 'way of seeing', is an important sociological contribution. It provides a wider insight into individual behaviour and social factors.

WHAT IS PSYCHOLOGY?

Psychology is the science of the brain and behaviour. It includes many sub-disciplines, some of which are relevant to medical education. For example, a focus of health psychology research is about behaviour change theories and interventions – this could be patient behaviour change, for example, around smoking cessation, or could be about health professional behaviour – increasing handwashing or a different patient referral route.

Psychology is the underpinning of many key concepts in medical education and medical education research – for example, problem-based learning.[4] Research in medical education has different themes in its development, with their roots in underpinning behavioural and social sciences – for example, reliability and validity of assessment.[5] In part, this focus is because psychologists and sociologists led the early waves in medical education research.[6]

To illustrate how sociology and psychology might help you, case studies from two different perspectives are discussed.

CASE STUDY FROM SOCIOLOGY: LEARNING STYLES, SOCIALITY AND HIDDEN CURRICULA
History

From a sociological perspective, learning is generally considered to be a social process taking place in a specific social context. This might be in terms of the sociality of learning, or the way that social factors impact and influence learning. The interest in sociality of learning is reflected in theories relevant to medical education research that sit at the edges of psychology such as social and sociocultural learning theories[7,8]. Interest in how social factors shape learning in medical education is reflected in the work on, for instance, how sexism impacts students.[9] There are also some critical concerns with the wider purposes and ways in which medical education works to reflect and build a sense of professional identity and structures of medical relationships and power.[10]

Focal concerns

Sociology has therefore looked at learning in medical education from a number of angles sometimes singly, predominantly one or another, or through a combination. It might imply:

- Examining or taking into account the sociology of the classroom. Understanding the roles, relationships of the classroom as a whole and also within a wider educational setting and asking, in what ways do these impact learning?

- Looking at differentials in learning experience, for instance in assessment, by sex, gender, age or sociodemographic background, knowing that each of these might impact performance.
- Taking into account or examining learning and teaching cultures. For instance, teacher and student preferences for asking and answering questions. This kind of research has repeatedly shown that young women ask fewer questions and are invited to answer questions less often than men in some learning contexts.[11]
- Concern with medical education as a process of acculturation into medicine as a profession, and therefore concerned with how medics model professional relationships and behaviour towards each other and towards patients, e.g. Bloom.[12]
- Understanding the 'hidden curriculum', comprising both informal learning from peers, but also the way that attitudes, values, beliefs and behaviours are promulgated in medical education.[10]

When applied to the issue of learning styles, these concerns can shift or complement a focus on the individual towards what influences how students learn from their experience, the environment and curriculum design.

Solution

When setting out to examine a specific learning experience in medical education, sociologists might ask what social factors, construed in ways outlined earlier, might be influential or impactful, on whom and in what ways. Rather than just come up with a method, they would look at what sociology has said about that relationship, what theories have been used to explain it and what methods of enquiry allow one to examine it.

This is a way of addressing what is sometimes pitched as a criticism of medical education research as 'theory-light' and, more positively, of recognising that using 'the sociological imagination' as a way into research in this field opens up pathways to being rigorous – linking through a practice and research process from intervention development and implementation to evaluation in ways that make it coherent, capable of ultimately 'speaking up' to theory and more academically credible.[13]

CASE STUDY FROM PSYCHOLOGY: LEARNING STYLES
History

Learning styles research has been carried out for over 50 years. Learning styles are defined as the way in which people like to learn, and what is most effective for them, for example, whether they are auditory, visual or kinaesthetic learners. This often makes intuitive sense to learners – for example, thinking about how they like to learn.

Concerns

While learners might have a preference for learning in a particular way, there is no robust research evidence that this has an effect on learner outcome.[14] Therefore, in 2002, the Organisation for Economic Co-operation and Development (OECD) declared learning styles a 'neuromyth'.[15] Since then, there have been numerous studies (over 500 on a PubMed search) about learning styles in medical education, suggesting that research about learning styles is still continuing.

Solution

By reading around the contemporary evidence outside of medical education, for example, in psychology,[16] the researcher might then consider other alternatives for investigating learners. In this instance, dual coding theory would be a good place to start.[17] See resources for a website about this.

IN CONCLUSION

By reading around the topic that you want to research, you can find out more about the underlying theories, and whether they are still used in those other fields. Reading in different fields often helps to develop your sociological and psychological imagination, and maybe see medical education in a different way. We would also advise approaching a sociologist or a psychologist as a collaborator. Not only might they be useful in pointing you towards relevant reading, they are also very good at methods and measures.

RESOURCES

The **British Psychological Society** produces a weekly, engaging, accessible email digest of new studies in psychology. These enable you to read a little about the latest studies in general psychology but give you ideas about the latest concepts and ideas. https://digest.bps.org.uk

Dual coding – very practical website to learn more about this. www.olicav.com

The **British Sociological Association** supports a large community of medical sociologists who run several study and regional groups and also stage an annual conference. You find more information here. https://www.britsoc.co.uk/groups/medical-sociology-groups/medical-sociology-medsoc-study-group/medsoc-groups/

There is also a **UK national network of Behavioural and Social Scientists who Teach in medicine (BeSST)** which can provide links and contacts to psychologists and sociologists who contribute to medical education and research. https://www.besst.info

A guide to **types of research in medical education** with some useful models https://www.researchgate.net/publication/51583224_'The_research_compass'_An_introduction_to_research_in_medical_education_AMEE_Guide_No_56/link/0a85e531917cb15086000000/download

REFERENCES

1. Mills CW. *The Sociological Imagination*. New York: Oxford University Press; 1959.
2. Goran D, Whitehead M. *Policies and Strategies to Promote Social Equity in Health*. Stockholm, Sweden; 1991.
3. Marmot M, Allen J, Goldblatt P, et al. *The Marmot Review: Fair Society, Healthy Lives*. London; 2010.
4. Norman G, Schmidt H. The psychological basis of problem-based learning: a review of the evidence. *Acad Med* 1992;67(9):557–565.
5. Rotgans JI. The themes, institutions, and people of medical education research 1988-2010: content analysis of abstracts from six journals. *Adv Health Sci Educ* 2012;17:515–527.
6. Norman G. Fifty years of medical education research: waves of migration. *Med Educ* 2011;45:785–791.
7. Bandura A, Walters RH. *Social learning theory*, Vol 1. Englewood Cliffs, NJ: Prentice Hall; 1977.
8. Vygotsky LS. *The Collected Works of LS Vygotsky*, Vol. 1. New York: Plenum Press. 1987:39–285.
9. Cheng L, Yang H. Learning about gender on campus: an analysis of the hidden curriculum for medical students. *Med Educ* 2015;49(3):321–331.
10. Hafferty FW, Castellani B. The hidden curriculum: a theory of medical education. In: Brosnan C, Turner BS, eds. *Handbook of the Sociology of Medical Education*. London: Routledge. 2009:15–36.
11. Carter AJ, Croft A, Lukas D, Sandstrom GM. Women's visibility in academic seminars: women ask fewer questions than men. *PLOS ONE* 2018;13(9):e0202743.
12. Bloom SW. The sociology of medical education: some comments on the state of a field. *Milbank Mem Fund Q* 1965;43(2):143–184.
13. Albert M. Understanding the debate on medical education research: a sociological perspective. *Acad Med* 2004;79(10):948–954.
14. Pashler H, McDaniel M, Rohrer D. Learning styles: concepts and evidence. *Psychol Sci Public Interes* 2009;9:105–119.
15. OECD. *Understanding the Brain: Towards a New Learning Science*. Paris: OECD. 2002.
16. Knoll AR, Otani H, Skeel RL, Van Horn KR. Learning style, judgements of learning, and learning of verbal and visual information. *Brit J Psychol* 2017;108(3):544–563.
17. Clark J, Paivio A. Dual coding theory and education. *Educ Psychol Rev* 1991;1(3):149–210.

CHAPTER 4

Co-creation and participatory processes in medical education research

Katrina F. Sawchuk and Vivian R. Ramsden

INTRODUCTION

Medical education research aims to advance the knowledge, skills and professionalism across the continuum of learners including patients.[1] Evaluating various aspects of learning and teaching is a fundamental part of everyone's job, every day, in all parts of the health care system. Thus, practical ways of answering questions that evolve from medical education in practice place importance on reflective practice. That said, questions that evolve can be answered using the appropriate suite of methods, to ultimately contribute to improved education, patient outcomes, practices and policies.[2]

One approach to answering questions that evolve from medical education could be mixed methods participatory social justice (MMPSJ). MMPSJ is an orientation that is framed within a construct of participatory processes or working *with* to co-create questions grounded in the virtues of knowledge reciprocity, relationship building and sustainability, commitment, participation and ultimately transformation.[3] This chapter uses the MMPSJ framework[4] as the guide to describe the use of participatory processes in each phase. The phases are outlined, followed by several reflective questions and an example.

APPLICATION OF PARTICIPATORY PROCESSES

Participatory processes often involve mixed methods which draw on strengths for both quantitative and qualitative research.[5] MMPSJ follows cyclical processes similar to action research. There have been four phases identified in the application of participatory processes.[4] These are as follows: identification of the problem; data collection undertaken by all members of the research team; analysis during which the research team connects the different data forms to build a stronger case for action/transformation and report the results in ways that can facilitate transformation.[4] What differentiates this methodology from others is that all members of the community, in this case learners, inclusive of patients and teachers are involved at every step, including the co-creation of the research question(s) and the issue(s) being addressed.

Some of the strengths of MMPSJ are identified as being appeal for all participants (learners, teachers and researchers), change and empowerment, all participants play an active role and researchers are facilitators guided by the participants throughout the processes.[6] By its nature, participatory work is relational, hence it takes a deep investment over time to build and sustain relationships.[6,7] Challenges in using new designs are as follows: having the necessary expertise so it is helpful to work with a participatory researcher;[8,9] co-creating a set of values prior to commencing the research project is critical to the building of mutual trust[10] and communicating what you have done to others so that the methods chosen need to be clearly outlined and documented as the participatory processes are applied throughout the phases.[11] Demonstrating humility and cultural competence when working with participants is crucial, but can also be a challenge.[12]

By involving participants in each phase, we honour and enrich all of our relationships. More importantly, the engagement should serve to engage the participants in empowering themselves in ways that are meaningful for them.

REFLECTIVE QUESTIONS

1. In what ways can medical education be developed? With whom can/should medical education be developed?
2. Where can ethical spaces[13] be created for data collection and knowledge translation?[14]
3. In what ways can diversity within the participants be recognised?

EXAMPLE

The social determinants of health[15] demonstrate that there is a different reality for people who live in poverty. Evidence indicated that one in nine adults in the Saskatoon Health Region[16] do not have a high school education which in turn impacts on their health and well-being; thus, this needs to be taken into consideration when developing educational materials for/with learners including patients, practitioners and researchers. The disparities are often grounded in historic power imbalances.[17] As learners, teachers, practitioners and researchers, we have a responsibility to address inequities in the community, e.g. opioid crises, Black Lives Matter, Indigenous Lives Matter. The why is evident, yet the how is often more complex. The MMPSJ framework puts forward the idea that by listening to the story and collaborating on every aspect of the process, e.g. data collection, analysis, results are meaningful and can transform the system.[4] In the following example, an Elder was invited to participate in co-creating connections between education and social determinants of health, which could then be used to co-create ways to increase the number of adults with a high school education.

> *'I grew up feeling the effects of colonization and that I was poor – that is a social engineered thing that the government created... but I can't say that I was poor compared to other contemporaries on the reserve. They had a hard time plus they had social ills like drinking, addictions, and depression ... all stemming from colonization. So I grew up as an anomaly; there are intergenerational effects of residential school affecting great grand parents, grandparents and children and epigenetically affecting Indigenous people at the cellular level. That's part of the problem out there; eventually we have to heal from a cellular level. Not heal from our anger but use our anger and hopefully that will help us to heal'* (Taken from transcript, 2019).[18] (Permission given by the Elder.)

GLOSSARY

- *Residential School*: In Canada, the Indigenous peoples have over a hundred years of experience with the residential school system. It was created for the purpose of eliminating Indigenous peoples as distinct and to assimilate them into Canadian mainstream against their will.[19]
- *Elder*: An Elder is a person recognised by a First Nation community as having knowledge and understanding of the traditional culture of the community, including the physical embodiment of the culture of the people and their spiritual and social traditions. Knowledge and wisdom, coupled with the recognition and respect of the people for their community, are the essential defining characteristics of an Elder. Some Elders have additional attributes, such as those of a traditional healer, or specialise in certain knowledge areas, such as education. Some Elders may also be specialists in certain histories and stories.

A TOOL FOR BUILDING SUCCESS

Consider applying the rubric in Table 4.1 for building success in using MMPSJ with your own educational research question(s). The fourth column has been left blank, as this is put forth both as a summary evolving from the previous elements, but also as a space for you to consider and position your research within MMPSJ. In this way, you will be able to see if your research question(s) aligns with MMPSJ. More importantly, co-creation attributes are highlighted for consideration.

TABLE 4.1 Rubric for applying MMPSJ in educational research

Creation Phase	Co-Creation Attributes	Intended Outcomes	Examples from Study
Identification of the problem.	Engage with the participants to co-create that which is meaningful to/for them.	Advocate for/with participants so that the research is seen as strength-based and inclusive.	
Data collection undertaken by all members of the research team including undergraduate medical students, residents and patients.	Use ways/strategies for engaging participants that focus on inclusivity.	Authentic engagement and sustainability of relationships over time.	
Analyses of the data collected by all of members of the research team.	Use different forms of data to build a case for action/ transformation.	Results/findings take into account all participants, e.g. undergraduate medical students and patients.	
Share the results/ findings that can facilitate action/ transformation.	Co-construct the results/findings to recognise and elucidate power relationships; translate the results/findings in ways that facilitate action transformation.	Enhance and build capacity; obtain funding when possible.	

SUMMARY/CONCLUSION

Medical education research aims to advance the knowledge, skills and professionalism across the continuum of learners including patients. By involving all participants in every phase, the outcomes will have meaning to all who were engaged in co-creating each of the phases.

REFERENCES

1. Association of American Medical Colleges. Research in medical education: a primer for medical students [Internet]. Washington, DC; 2015. 16 p. Available from: https://www.aamc.org/system/files/c/2/429856-mededresearchprimer.pdf.
2. Hosain J, Reis O, Verrall T, et al. Grounded in practice: integrating practice improvement into daily activities. *Can Fam Physician*. 2020 Dec; 66(12):931–933.
3. Mertens DM. Transformative paradigm: mixed methods and social justice. *J Mix Methods Res* 2007 Jul;1(3):212–225.
4. Creswell JW, Piano Clark VL. *Designing and Conducting Mixed Methods Research.* 3rd ed. Thousand Oaks, CA: Sage Publications; 2018:492 p.
5. Johnson RB, Onwuegbuzie AJ. Mixed methods research: a research paradigm whose time has come. *Educ Res* 2004;33(7):14–26.
6. Ramsden VR, Crowe J, Rabbitskin N, Rolfe D, Macaulay AC. Chapter 6: authentic engagement, co-creation and action research. In: Goodyear-Smith F, Mash B, eds. *How To Do Primary Care Research.* Boca Raton, FL: CRC Press; 2019: 47–56.
7. Allen ML, Salsberg J, Knot M, et al. Engaging with communities, engaging with patients: amendment to the NAPCRG 1998 Policy Statement on Responsible Research with Communities. *Fam Pract* 2017 Jun 1;34(3):313–321. doi:10.1093/fampra/cmw074.
8. Ramsden VR, Integrated Primary Health Care Research Team. Learning with the community: evolution to transformative action research. *Can Fam Physician* 2003 Feb;49(2):195–197, 200–202.
9. Martin R, Chan R, Torikka L, Granger-Brown A, Ramsden V. Health fostered by research. *Can Fam Physician* 2008 Feb;54(2):244–245.
10. Ramsden VR, McKay S, Crowe J. The pursuit of excellence: engaging the community in participatory health research. *Glob Health Promot* 2010 Dec;17(4):32–42. doi:10.1177/1757975910383929.
11. Ivankova N, Wingo N. Applying mixed methods in action research: methodological potentials and advantages. *Am Behav Sci* 2018 Jun;62(7):978–997.
12. Isaacson M. Clarifying concepts: cultural humility or competency. *J Prof Nurses* 2014 May;30(3):251–258.
13. Ermine W. The ethical space of engagement. *Indig Law J* 2007;6(1):193–203.
14. Nguyen T, Graham ID, Mrklas K, et al. How does integrated knowledge translation (IKT) compare to other collaborative research approaches to generating and translating knowledge? Learning from experts in the field. *Health Res Policy Sys* 2020;18(1):35. doi:10.1186/s12961-020-0539-6.
15. Commission on Social Determinants of Health. *Closing the gap in a generation: health equity through action on the social determinants of health. Final Report of the Commission on Social Determinants of Health.* Geneva, Switzerland: World Health Organization; 2008.
16. Saskatoon Health Region. Community view collaboration: building evidence for action. Available from: https://www.communityview.ca/infographic_SHR_determinants.html.

17. Truth and Reconciliation Commission of Canada. *Truth and Reconciliation Commission of Canada: Calls to Action.* Winnipeg, MN: National Centre for Truth and Reconciliation; 2015.

18. Kanewivakiho, D Elder, Sawchuk KF, Ramsden VR. Ask before you ask: co-developing meaningful questions with Indigenous Elders. *Canadian Family Physician.* Under review.

19. Kaspar V. The lifetime effect of residential school attendance on indigenous health status. *Am J Public Health* 2014 Nov;104(11):2184–2190.

CHAPTER 5

Educational research and policymaking

John Yaphe

Primary care medicine faces challenges as a profession and educational research can help the disciplines involved to cope with these challenges. This chapter reviews some recent educational research in primary care and describes how it has influenced policy. It is based on remarks from the Janko Kersnik memorial lecture at the second EURACT educational research conference held in Leuven in 2018.

The 'Five C's' traditionally characterise primary care. These are continuous, comprehensive, context-based care, coordinated by the primary care team with other levels of care, and characterised by excellent communication between health care professionals and patients. All of these elements have been the subject of research, but more research is needed, as styles and structures of practice change. These changes will influence the ways we teach our students and trainees and how we manage lifelong learning.

For example, continuity of care as a value continues to be challenged, as new models of practice emerge.[1] In place of a single provider giving 24-hour care, we now have team-based models of practice in many places, with organisational continuity of the team or of the medical record, without adverse effects on patient outcomes.[2] As we describe these changes in our research and assess their outcomes, we need to change the ways we teach this value to our learners.

There are five new Cs that I would like to propose as the agenda for future educational research, and explore the ways that this will affect educational policy in medicine. The first C refers to financial constraints, found in all health systems. The second refers to computers and the influence of information overload on practice. The computer is also a source of interference in provider-patient communication. We need to teach the rational use of this tool to our students, trainees and colleagues in practice. The third C refers to confidentiality. Ethical issues are challenged by informatics. The fourth refers to complexity and uncertainty as inevitable factors in medical practice. Practicing medicine 'at the edge of chaos' has policy implications on how we teach this subject. The fifth C stands for corrosion, a synonym for burnout. Research on this topic suggests that there is a need for policy changes in all-educational institutions involved in the teaching and training of health professionals.

The challenges we face lie in adapting principles enunciated over 50 years ago, when family medicine/general practice (GP) was created as an academic discipline, to a changed world. This chapter presents examples from recent educational research, and explores how this has influenced educational policy.

CONTEXT

We need to teach our learners in the context in which they will practice. We no longer have the luxury of dividing undergraduate medical education into preclinical and clinical subjects, because everything is clinical. If an educational topic has no relevance for the benefit of patients, then it has no place in the curriculum. An influential study by members of EURACT Council mapped the rise of early clinical exposure courses in Europe.[3] Almost 80% of the universities surveyed had early clinical exposure for their students in the first years of their medical studies. Since the study was published in 2009, it has been cited over 50 times. Subsequent research has demonstrated the value of this method.[4] Almost all medical schools in Europe now probably provide direct contact with patients for their medical students, though the current coronavirus crisis has hindered this process. Increasing number of schools will do this under the direction of primary care tutors in community clinics. This is a positive example of research changing policy.

There is a need for a move from traditional medical education that tends to be frontal, hierarchical, passive and dogmatic to active, self-directed learning in context. A mixed methods study using qualitative and quantitative research methods involving medical students and their GP teachers explored what medical students want.[5] Our students value active learning in a friendly environment, seeing patients as people, learning practical skills with a variety of teaching methods and receiving timely feedback from enthusiastic teachers. The provision of more GP education in the undergraduate curriculum in many medical schools is recognition of these learning needs. Systematic reviews have shown how family medicine teaching has had positive effects in many settings.[6] These principles can also be applied in vocational training. Disciplines outside primary care are also using the methods of modern adult education in the training of young specialists in many fields.

FINANCIAL CONSTRAINTS

The challenge of coping with financial constraints has been addressed in educational research. This research needs to be translated into practical lessons with patients. A study of the ways that primary care doctors cope with conflicts over health insurance issues was a step in this direction.[7] This analysis of coping patterns has been incorporated into teaching programmes on doctor-patient communication for undergraduate and postgraduate students, and learners in continuing education, with some success.[8] Financial issues cannot be left to the managers. Involving medical professionals and patients in the resolution of these issues requires a proactive change in policy regarding the ways we teach this subject.

ASSESSMENT

A change in policy is also required regarding the ways we assess learning. Educational research can help us in this area. Oral examinations have been a traditional form of assessment in medicine, especially in high-stakes situations. They have their unique qualities; however, they are also plagued by difficulties with validity and reliability. A study of decision-making among oral examiners in college examinations in GP in the United Kingdom provided a fascinating look into the minds of examiners.[9] The findings of this study have helped to change examination policy to make for fairer, more valid and more reliable assessments. However, feedback to examiners does not always help them to get it right.[10] There are implications here for assessment at the undergraduate, postgraduate and continuing education levels.

TEACHING RESEARCH

Teaching our students, trainees and colleagues in practice to do research can also be a powerful tool in their education. Training in research does not universally occur in undergraduate student, vocational trainee or practitioner medical education, hence a change in policyis also required. Recent examples of published medical student research show how our students can lead the way towards policy change by asking the right questions. Research on excessive prescription of psychotropic drugs[11] and the use of placebos in GP[12] can lead to changes in practice to benefit patients. We need to study the effects of research training on the careers of our learners. This can help to promote the research agenda in medical education at all levels. There are effective ways to help our motivated learners to engage in research.[13]

Society is changing, and primary care medicine is changing along with it. Can we change our educational objectives, methods and assessment to meet the changing needs of our patients, our learners and our profession? Timely, accurate research can shape our teaching programmes. I encourage our educators to maintain a critical view of their work and to continue on this path.

REFERENCES

1. Yaphe, J. Continuity of care: a changing value as time goes by. *Revista Portuguesa de Medicina Geral e Familiar* 2013;29:358–359.
2. Parkerton PH, Smith DG, Straley HL. Primary care practice coordination versus physician continuity. *Fam Med* 2004;36(1):15–21.
3. Başak O, Yaphe J, Spiegel W, Wilm S, Carelli F, Metsemakers JFM. Early clinical exposure in medical curricula across Europe: an overview. *Eur J Gen Pract* 2009;15:4–10.
4. Wenrich MD, Jackson MB, Wolfhagen I, Ramsey PG, Scherpbier AJ. What are the benefits of early patient contact?–A comparison of three preclinical patient contact settings. *BMC Med Educ* 2013;13:80.
5. Snadden D, Yaphe J. General practice and medical education: what do medical students value? *Med Teach* 1996;18:31–34.
6. Turkeshi E, Michels NR, Hendrickx K, et al. Impact of family medicine clerkships in undergraduate medical education: a systematic review. *BMJ Open*2015;5:e008265.
7. Weingarten MA, Guttman N, Abramovitch H, et al. An anatomy of conflicts in primary care encounters: a multi-method study. *Fam Pract* 2010;27:93–100.
8. Walter A, Chew-Graham C, Harrison S. Negotiating refusal in primary care consultations: a qualitative study. *Fam Pract* 2012;29(4):488–496.
9. Yaphe J, Street S. How do examiners decide? A qualitative study of the process of decision making in the oral examination component of the MRCGP examination. *Med Educ* 2003;37:764–771.
10. Sturman N, Ostini R, Wong WY, Zhang J, David M. "On the same page"? The effect of GP examiner feedback on differences in rating severity in clinical assessments: a pre/post intervention study. *BMC Med Educ* 2017;17(1):101.
11. Lopes R., Yaphe J., Ribas M. Psychotropic medication prescribing in primary care in Porto: a cross-sectional study. *Revista Portuguesa de Medicina Geral e Familiar* 2014;30:368–376.
12. Braga-Simões J, Soares Costa P, Yaphe J. Placebo prescription and empathy of the physician: a cross-sectional study. *Eur J Gen Pract* 2017;23:98–104.
13. Marais DL, Kotlowitz J, Willems B, Barsdorf NW, van Schalkwyk S. Perceived enablers and constraints of motivation to conduct undergraduate research in a Faculty of Medicine and Health Sciences: what role does choice play? *PLOS ONE* 2019;14(3):e0212873.

CHAPTER 6

Scope and research environment

Roger Strasser

> We need high-quality medical education research to help us
> ensure our educational practice is theoretically sound; to develop
> approaches to the problems that matter in primary care education;
> and to inform sane policy.[1]

Primary care education is about context, specifically people living in their
local home/family/community context.[2] This contrasts with most health
workforce education, particularly medical education, that is based implicitly
on the notion that discipline knowledge and skills are context independent
or 'objective'. The reality is that most clinical education occurs in large
urban teaching hospitals, so most medical education research is set in those
environments.[3] In addition, the principal clinical teachers and mentors for
medical students are medical discipline specialists or subspecialists who view
their field of medicine as pre-eminent and superior to other fields, particularly
primary care.[4] This perspective is often identified as part of the 'hidden
curriculum' of medical education.[5] The paradox of the predominance of
teaching hospitals in medical education is that 21st-century teaching hospitals
have a highly selected patient population; generally, individuals who are
extremely sick have rare diseases or require specific high-tech interventions.[6]
In addition, patients' lengths of stay in teaching hospitals are often very short,
which further limits educational opportunities for students and trainees, as
well as opportunities for educational research.

Around the world, there are many forms and styles of primary care, with
variations between countries and within countries reflecting variations in

geography, demography, language, culture, sociology and climate, as well as economic, social and educational status of the population. In addition, the health system and how health services are funded varies from country to country. Primary care may be delivered principally by medical practitioners (with or without formal general practice/family medicine training), solo or in groups, or by other health workers including community health workers and nurses, or by teams of health care providers. Despite all these variations, primary care is always local care focussed on addressing the health needs of the population being served.[7-9] This dimension of local context, often referred to as 'place', provides wonderful opportunities for educational and clinical experiences for students and trainees, coupled with the challenge of ensuring and enhancing the quality and effectiveness of these experiences. This challenge highlights the exciting potential and the broad scope of primary care educational research (PCER).

Relationships are central to high-quality primary care and a key feature of primary care education.[9,10] There is a strong parallel process between the patient-doctor relationship and the learner-teacher relationship. Paul Worley identified four principal relationship dimensions in his symbiotic medical education system (Figure 6.1) that was based on his study of the Parallel Rural Community Curriculum (PRCC), in which medical students

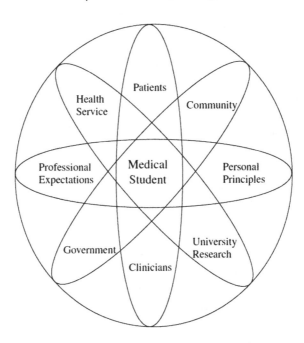

FIGURE 6.1 The symbiotic medical education system.

Source: Worley P, Prideaux D, Strasser, et al. Empirical evidence for symbiotic medical education: a comparative analysis of community and tertiary-based programmes. *Med Edu* 2006;40:109–116.

learn their core clinical medicine during a year based in rural general practice.[11] With the medical student in the centre, these relationships are patients-clinicians, community-government, personal-professional and university-health service, and all are connected within the circle of context. These relationship dimensions add richness to primary care education and expand opportunities for PCER. Longitudinal Integrated Clerkships (LICs) like the PRCC, particularly in rural primary care, add the dimension of community immersion, whereby students and trainees are living and learning in communities for prolonged periods of time.[12-14] Putting all these dimensions together, the possibilities for PCER are almost limitless. PCER is certainly much more than studies of teaching techniques in the primary care setting.

With limitless possibilities, why is PCER relatively uncommon and underrepresented in medical education research? For primary care providers, there are many practical barriers to PCER, like lack of dedicated time, administrative support and space. However, the most formidable obstacle is a mindset issue. Many primary care providers do not see themselves as educators, let alone researchers. In their minds, education is lectures and ward rounds (which they do not do) and research is undertaken by specialists (in the extreme wearing white coats and holding test tubes), so they are neither educators nor researchers.[15,16] As mentioned already, there is a strong parallel process between patient-doctor relationships and the learner-teacher relationships, so in fact experienced primary care providers have substantial educational skills developed through their interactions with patients.[17] Similarly, daily interactions with patients raise questions which frequently are answered by consulting the literature or a colleague; however, occasionally, there is no answer and potentially this is the beginning of a research project.

There are many possible sources of PCER research questions, beginning with learner-teacher interactions around specific patients or clinical problems that may spark research into how students and trainees learn about the clinical problem, and how to interact with patients with that problem. One day, a colleague in rural family practice was surprised when the patient asked, *'where is the student?'* The colleague was surprised because he had seen the presence of medical students as something of an imposition on patients, but he enjoyed teaching. In this case, the patient went on to explain that, when there is a student present, the doctor asks questions and shares more information which is beneficial to the patient as well as the student. This interaction could be the beginning of a study of patients' perceptions and expectations of students in primary care education; or it could be a study of how primary care providers could involve patients in teaching; or it could be a study of students' perception of learning with and from patients.

To help move past the mindset obstacle, it is important to realise that there are many ways to make a start in PCER, and that there are many sources of support, guidance and assistance in undertaking PCER. For example, departments of primary care/general practice/family medicine have expertise and provide access to courses on many aspects of education and of research. Internationally, the World Organization of Family Doctors (WONCA) provides many resources online.[18] The courses may be short courses accessed through continuing professional development or university graduate studies in the form of Graduate Certificates, Graduate Diplomas, Masters or PhDs. Increasingly, these courses are accessible asynchronously online so that primary care providers can learn the skills of educational research without having to travel to the academic institution and at the most convenient times for them. There is no substitute for discussion with colleagues, staff, learners and patients in exploring potential research questions and developing specific studies. Participation in online courses often includes specific projects or assignments which encourage and support these collegial discussions in developing education research skills.

As you explore the potential of PCER, the many dimensions of primary care education open a wide range of aspects of potential studies. Of course, there is research in the primary care context about enhancing the quality and effectiveness of clinical teaching by the primary care educators and staff, other learners, patients and the broader community whether this is one-on-one teaching, small group learning or addressing particular clinical topics. There is also research focussed on key aspects of primary care like the patient-doctor relationship, clinical decision-making, adaptive expertise and social accountability. In addition, one study may lead to another. This has been my experience over the years. For example, an ongoing study tracking medical students and trainees of the Northern Ontario School of Medicine (NOSM) in Canada continues to focus on specialty choice and practice location of graduates, but also has opened questions about how students learn.[19,20] Interviews of students as they began their studies and at graduation opened insights about their perspective on family practice in rural settings that lead to further interviews of graduates in family practice to complete a study of NOSM students and graduates experience of generalism in rural practice.[21] These findings opened questions about how students learn generalism skills that now contribute to research into learning adaptive expertise.

Another example from my experience relates to the NOSM LIC in which medical students learn their core clinical medicine living and learning in 1 of 15 communities across Northern Ontario based in family practice. This line of research began with exploring the students' experience of the transitions from classroom learner to clinician during the academic year,[22] and opened questions about the contribution of communities in the professional identity formation of the students.[23]

As I have described, PCER has many dimensions and possibilities limited only by our own imagination. As you launch into PCER, the only source of fear is fear itself. Now is the time to participate and contribute to truly innovative and creative PCER, specifically *research in primary care, about primary care education* that presents the importance and enhances the value of primary care education. This PCER may just contribute to achieving Marshall Marinker's bold aspiration for general practice and academic medicine.

> I believe that the task of general practice in the medical school is to reconstruct the discipline of medicine, to make coherent and whole what modern technology has shattered[24]

REFERENCES

1. Peile E. Parting thoughts on medical education research and education for primary care. *Educ Prim Care* 2014;25(6):297–298.
2. Howe A. Has a decade made a difference? The contribution of UK primary care to basic medical training in 2004. *Educ Prim Care* 2005;16(1):10–19.
3. Prislin MD, Saultz JW, Geyman JP. The generalist disciplines in American medicine one hundred years following the Flexner Report: a case study of unintended consequences and some proposals for post-Flexnerian reform. *Acad Med* 2010;85:228–235.
4. Frenk J, Chen L, Bhutta ZA, et al. Health professionals for a new century: transforming education to strengthen health systems in an interdependent world. *Lancet* 2010;376(9756):1923–1958.
5. Hafferty FW. Beyond curriculum reform: confronting medicine's hidden curriculum. *Acad Med* 1998;73:403–407.
6. Green L, Fryer G, Yawn B, et al. The ecology of medical care revisited. *N Engl J Med* 2001;344(26):2021–2025.
7. Starfield B, Shi L, Macinko J. Contribution of primary care to health systems and health. *Milbank Q* 2005;83:457–502.
8. Van Weel C, Howe A. *Primary Health Care around the World: Recommendations for International Policy and Development.* Boca Raton, FL: CRC Press, Taylor & Francis Group; 2019.
9. McWhinney IR. *A Textbook of Family Medicine.* Oxford, UK: Oxford University Press; 1989.
10. Stewart M, Brown JB, Weston W, et al. *Patient-Centred Medicine: Transforming the Clinical Method.* Boca Raton, FL: CRC Press, Taylor & Francis Group; 2014.
11. Worley P, Prideaux D, Strasser, et al. Empirical evidence for symbiotic medical education: a comparative analysis of community and tertiary-based programmes. *Med Educ* 2006;40:109–116.
12. Strasser R, Worley P, Cristobal F, et al. Putting communities in the driver's seat: the realities of community engaged medical education. *Acad Med* 2015;90:1466–1470.
13. Strasser R, Hogenbirk J, Jacklin K, et al. Community engagement: a central feature of NOSM's socially accountable distributed medical education. *Can Med Educ J* 2018;9(1):e33–e43.

14. Strasser R. Students learning medicine in general practice in Canada and Australia. *Aust Fam Physician* 2016;45(1–2):22–25.
15. Hennen BK. The dragon research. *Can Fam Physician* 1988;34:1265–1417.
16. Ventres W, Whiteside-Mansell L. Getting started in research, redefined: five questions for clinically focused physicians in family medicine. *Fam Med Com Health* 2019;7:e000017.
17. Miflin B, Price D. Rural doctors are naturally effective teachers. *Aust J Rural Health* 1993;2(1):21–28.
18. WONCA. The World Organization of Family Doctors. 2020. Available from: https://www.globalfamilydoctor.com/
19. Hogenbirk JC, French MG, Timony PE, et al. Outcomes of the Northern Ontario School of Medicine's distributed medical education programmes: protocol for a longitudinal comparative multicohort study. *BMJ Open* 2015;5(7):e008246.
20. Hogenbirk JC, Timony P, French MG, et al. Milestones on the Social Accountability Journey: family medicine practice locations of Northern Ontario School of Medicine graduates. *Can Fam Physician* 2016;62:e138–e145.
21. Strasser R, Cheu H. The needs of the many: NOSM students' experience of generalism and rural practice. *Can Fam Physician* 2018;64:449–455.
22. Dube TV, Schinke RJ, Strasser R, et al. Transition processes through a longitudinal integrated clerkship: a qualitative study of medical students' experiences. *Med Educ* 2015;49:1028–1037.
23. Dube TV, Schinke RJ, Strasser R. It takes a community to train a future physician: social support experienced by medical students during a community-engaged longitudinal integrated clerkship. *Can Med Edu J* 2019;10(3):e55–e60.
24. Marinker M. The chameleon, the Judas goat, and the cuckoo. *J R Coll Gen Pract* 1978;28:199–206.

CHAPTER 7

Integrating primary and secondary care educational research

Hélène Elidor

Although levels of health care matter for organisational structure and care delivery purposes, few health care challenges respect disciplinary boundaries.[1] Indeed, research, that takes into account the holistic nature of societal problems by integrating training, understanding and knowledge from different levels of care, is essential to finding innovative solutions to health problems.[2] Primary and secondary care professionals, whether in the public or private sector, need to learn together, cooperatively seeking solutions to the challenges of our time, so that together they can create a more sustainable health care system.[3,4] The need for collaborative health care educational research is particularly important for quality improvement, efficient health care delivery and patient-centred practice.[5] However, literature on collaborative work shows that generalists and specialists tend to be grouped around their specific disciplinary, academic or field interests.[2] This chapter puts into perspective the importance of integrating primary with secondary care educational research.

First, we need to define integrated educational research. One definition is the process of facilitating and incorporating learning or knowledge through careful consideration of disciplines involved in addressing a particular concern to achieve the common goal of producing new scientific knowledge.[5,6] Integrated educational research is especially relevant for achieving advances in health care towards collaborative interprofessional working. We consider primary and secondary care professionals as two separate disciplines. Interacting together to learn and investigate around specific questions allows them to improve their knowledge, skills and habits regarding the delivery of care to the user.

> 'To understand the world, it has seemed necessary to analyse it by breaking it into many pieces (ie, the disciplines and their own divisions). But to act in the world, to try to address the issues for the understanding of which highly specialized knowledge was presumably sought, we need to somehow reassemble all the pieces. ... put our knowledge together again for coping with the whole real problems of the world'.[7,8]

Traditionally, generalists tend to provide primary and community care, whereas secondary care tends to be provided by specialists, most often in the hospital. While generalists used to have education training in hospital, the opposite is not necessarily true for specialists.[9] Along the same lines, primary and secondary care educational research has independent focus, making collaborative work more difficult and reinforcing the fragmented care delivery at the expense of best practices; however, efforts to address these shortcomings are needed and timely, in view of opportunities for mutual understanding of health care challenges, broader knowledge and educational innovation, which is necessary to ultimately improve health outcomes for all (Table 7.1).

PROMOTING MUTUAL UNDERSTANDING AND A COMMON GOAL

Integrating educational research is an approach to improving the understanding of complex and real-world problems by analysing a question from various points of view. Mutual learning seeks to bring together methods and insights from each individual field to resolve a specific question. As a result, it challenges generalists and specialists to move beyond the uniqueness of their field by connecting ideas, beliefs and concepts across different field boundaries.[9] Furthermore, learning together facilitates interprofessional relationships which are widely encouraged in collaborative work,[12] and essential in research where mutual understanding and trust are paramount.

MORE IN-DEPTH TOPIC COVERAGE

Research is tough work. We know how daunting it can be to plan meaningful questions, collect unbiased data and build convincing arguments. Researchers often need more than one reason to explain their result or claim. Doing research in collaboration with others can bring in-depth understanding, more comprehensive knowledge and additional value. Integrated research learning presents opportunities to solve previously intractable problems for each discipline in its own way or in silos.[13] This type of learning helps to better tackle complex problems more in depth.

TABLE 7.1 Characteristics of primary care, secondary care and integrating primary care educational research with secondary care educational research

	Participants' Discipline	Research Style/ Focus	Examples from Literature
Primary care	From primary care	Engage patients/ communities Integrate innovations into practice Seek best way to organise care to meet the needs of the population	How does small group continuing medical education impact practice for rural GPs and their patients? Dowling et al.[10]
Secondary care	From secondary care	Determine treatment benefits/efficacy Identify best way to manage specific disease	What are treatment benefits for chronic diseases such as hypertension? Hare et al.[11]
Integrating primary with secondary care research	From both primary and secondary care	Engage generalists and specialists Determine ways to apply best treatment in community context	How could generalists and specialists learn more together? Spicer and Roberts[2]

BETTER MANAGEMENT OF CHRONIC DISEASES

Multiple chronic conditions are common, and there is increased worldwide concern to address the growing burden resulting from them. In addition, the prevalence of chronic diseases is increasing as the global life expectancy rises around the world.[14] As a result, more people are expected to have more than one disease requiring long-term prevention and management from both primary care physicians and other specialists. Linking primary and secondary educational research is a promising approach to responding to the burden of multiple chronical conditions. Health care systems are complex, unequal and most often fragmented. Learning together can bridge boundaries between generalists and specialists, shape successful collaborations and overcome complexities of health care systems.

Let us consider educational research aimed at identifying ways to implement innovations to manage patients suffering from a specific chronic disease, such as rheumatoid arthritis, a systemic, inflammatory disorder with a significant impact on the patients' quality of life.[15] While secondary care researchers focus on identifying the most effective treatment, primary care researchers may want to know more about pragmatic ways to provide social support, improve therapeutic adherence and the patients' quality of life or involve patients and caregivers in the research. Both points of view are legitimate and important. Both generalists and specialists may conduct randomised control trials, make causal inference from observational data or use other methods to collect quantitative or qualitative data or both; however, separated in silos, research remains fragmented around the disease. By working together, generalists and specialists can explore how best to manage the disease by integrating these two perspectives for the benefit of patients, their families and best practices. Joint learning is the key to facilitating the delivery of integrated care and maximising outcomes in the treatment of people with significant chronic conditions.

Integrated educational research approaches are needed to address the most complex and critical health care challenges facing health care systems today, including the prevention and management of chronic diseases. A key consideration in integrated learning is the nature of the research partnerships that are formed and the potential of future collaboration. Generalists and specialists learn with, about and from one another which maximises their individual contribution to a higher level. This interactive learning creates a powerful catalyst for supportive and productive cooperation. For the sake of the patients they treat, the sustainability of the health care system they support and the best practices they cherish, it is more important than ever that generalists and specialists join forces, learning from common ground to achieve a higher purpose and more effective care.

REFERENCES

1. Edwards ST, Hooker ER, Brienza R, et al. Association of a multisite interprofessional education initiative with quality of primary care. *JAMA Netw Open* 2019;2(11):e1915943.
2. Spicer J, Roberts R. Teaching and learning at the primary-secondary care interface: work in progress? *Educ Prim Care* 2020. 31(3):1–4.
3. Frenk J, Chen L, Bhutta ZA, et al. Health professionals for a new century: transforming education to strengthen health systems in an interdependent world. *Lancet* 2010;376(9756):1923–1958.
4. Nicholson C, Jackson C, Marley J. A governance model for integrated primary/secondary care for the health-reforming first world–results of a systematic review. *BMC Health Serv Res* 2013;13(1):528.
5. Mertens F, de Groot E, Meijer L, et al. Workplace learning through collaboration in primary healthcare: a BEME realist review of what works, for whom and in what circumstances: BEME guide no. 46. *Med Teach* 2018;40(2):117–134.
6. Green BN, Johnson CD. Interprofessional collaboration in research, education, and clinical practice: working together for a better future. *J Chiropr Educ* 2015;29(1):1–10.
7. Easton D, Schelling CS. *Divided Knowledge: Across Disciplines, Across Cultures.* Sage Publications: Newbury Park, USA. 1991.

8. Easton D. The division, integration, and transfer of knowledge. *Bull Am Acad Arts Sci* 1991. 44(4):8–27.

9. King N, Bravington A, Brooks J, et al. "Go make your face known": collaborative working through the lens of personal relationships. *Int J Integr Care* 2017;17(4):3. DOI: 10.5334/ijic.2574

10. Dowling S, Last J, Finnegan H, et al. How does small group continuing medical education (CME) impact on practice for rural GPs and their patients, a mixed-methods study. *Educ Prim Care* 2020:31(3): 153–161.

11. Hare JM, Bolli R, Cooke JP, et al. Phase II clinical research design in cardiology: learning the right lessons too well: observations and recommendations from the Cardiovascular Cell Therapy Research Network (CCTRN). *Circulation* 2013;127(15):1630–1635.

12. Pullon S. Competence, respect and trust: key features of successful interprofessional nurse-doctor relationships. *J Interprof Care* 2008;22(2):133–147.

13. Witteman HO, Stahl JE, Group ISiHC. Facilitating interdisciplinary collaboration to tackle complex problems in health care: report from an exploratory workshop. *Health Syst* 2013;2(3):162–170.

14. Organization WH. Life expectancy increased by 5 years since 2000, but health inequalities persist. World Health Statistics; 2016.

15. Tugwell P, Bombardier C, Buchanan WW, et al. Methotrexate in rheumatoid arthritis: impact on quality of life assessed by traditional standard-item and individualized patient preference health status questionnaires. *Arch Intern Med* 1990;150(1):59–62.

CHAPTER 8

Primary care interprofessional educational research

Robin Miller,
Nynke Scherpbier and
Peter Pype

INTRODUCTION

Interprofessional collaboration has always been a feature of primary care, but its importance has become emphasised over recent years as a vital component of an effective, efficient and sustainable health and care system.[1] This recognition is due to multiple factors, including ageing populations, changing social contexts, increased people with multiple long-term conditions, expectations from patients that they will be more involved in decisions, financial pressures on health and care services and the deployment of new digital technologies. Despite its long-term engagement with interprofessional working, there remain many challenges to primary care achieving collaboration consistently in practice.[2] Barriers exist at all levels of the system including those of policy, finance, regulation and organisations.[3] There is though considerable evidence that professionals do not always demonstrate the underlying values, skills and behaviours that are necessary to collaborate successfully with those from different professions.[4,5] The introduction of new roles and blurring of traditional professional boundaries are adding further complexities.

One approach to facilitating better collaboration within primary care is interprofessional education (IPE). This seeks to break down barriers through providing a safe learning environment in which professionals and students can address knowledge gaps of their respective expertise and responsibilities, challenge established stereotypes and misunderstandings and facilitate the development of greater respect and trust. Interest in IPE is long-standing with an international body (Centre for the Advancement of Interprofessional Education) to promote its practice established in 1987 and its endorsement by the World Health Organization.[1] There remains, however, a degree of scepticism that it must be a central component of pre- and post-registration programmes in health and social care, and it is often sidelined, rather than embedded fully in core curriculums. There are many reasons for this position, including the practical challenges of bringing together cohorts of learners from different professions, already crowded curriculums within professional training programmes and educators not always feeling confident in overseeing its design and delivery.[6–9]

This chapter begins by outlining current knowledge of IPE in primary care, and considering the challenges and opportunities of undertaking research in this area of educational practice.

IPE WITHIN PRIMARY CARE

IPE is defined as 'students from two or more professions learn about, from and with each other to enable effective collaboration and improve health outcomes'.[1] It has been successfully introduced within undergraduate, postgraduate and continuing professional development (CPD) education. IPE in pre-qualification programmes often considers general collaboration skills between professions in health and social care such as team working, whereas in post-qualification it is commonly deployed in relation to improving care for a particular population or condition, and/or to support an improvement programme within primary care. IPE draws upon group and active-based educational methods used within other professional teaching programmes including simulations, community-based projects, joint assessment and support for patients and families and e-learning.[6] The European Forum for Primary Care has published a position statement on IPE. Based on interprofessional workshops and an evidence review, this identifies common enablers of good practice across the undergraduate, postgraduate and CPD programmes (Table 8.1).[9] There is stronger evidence at present regarding positive impact on learner-focussed outcomes such as improved attitudes and perceptions of other professionals, and increased collaborative knowledge and skills.[8] There is still limited evidence to date of changes in professional behaviour and improved outcomes for patients and their families.

RESEARCH AND IPE

Researching IPE involves similar issues to that of studies of uni-professional education but with added complexities. Similar to primary care professionals, most researchers are specialists in their own discipline and steeped in related concepts, evidence based and preferred methodologies. They are

TABLE 8.1 Enablers of IPE in primary care[9]

Enabler	Related Activities
Involved patients	Patient stories shared within programme, joint home visits by students, co-design with patients, patient-led learning
Holistic focus	Multi-professional assessments of patient and families, emphasis on patient experience, exploration of determinants of health
Practical orientation	Arranging direct support for patients and families, learners undertaking shared project, community action to respond to health inequality
Multimodal	Shared lectures, online learning platforms, group discussions, team tasks, collective reflections, observation of interprofessional collaborative practice
Multi-professional	More than two professions, disciplines within profession, multiple agencies involved in coordination and design, public, voluntary and private sectors
Robust evaluation	Outcomes defined at outset of programme, formative and summative design, range of impacts considered including patients, communities, learners, and organisations, mixed methodologies
Team based	Learners undertaking practical group projects, team learning tasks, opportunities for shared reflection

often most comfortable in furthering knowledge in familiar contexts and the parameters, norms and restrictions that these contain. By its nature, IPE requires engagement with other academic groups who will have a different set of interests, research cultures and bodies of knowledge. Alongside such interdisciplinary complexities, there are other complications relating to the study of IPE in primary care. On a practical note, whilst IPE is embedded on a long-term basis in some educational programmes at pre- and post-registration, there is a tendency for IPE to be introduced on a short-term pilot basis. Long-term sustainability is then dependent on a few local academics and practice individuals who champion its benefits. This is a challenge for research, as such uncertainty makes robust design more difficult and in particular to not only investigate learning outcomes but to investigate the ultimate goal: outcomes for patients and families.

Despite all these challenges, there is an established tradition of IPE research. Primary care is well-represented alongside that relating to generic professional pre-registration courses and post-registration/CPD programmes within hospital settings.[9] Over the last two decades, there has been a steady increase in the number of studies published through specialist journals such as the Journal of Interprofessional Care, and generic health and care educational journals. For example, a Best Evidence Medical Education (BEME) Collaboration review undertaken in 2007, and then repeated in 2016, found that there was an increase from 21 to 46 high-quality studies that met the standard for inclusion.[8] The majority of published IPE studies are undertaken in Europe, USA, Canada and Australia. Research has largely focussed on IPE involving doctors and nurses and how they interact with other professions, with some professions being represented infrequently.[10,11]

Over time, common approaches are promoted within IPE research to help with consistency and comparability. These include – evaluation frameworks (e.g. the '3-P' model),[12] outcome frameworks (e.g. the IPE adapted Kirkpatrick model)[13] and validated tools (e.g. readiness for interprofessional learning [RIPLS][14]; see Box 8.1 for an example within primary research). Reviews have though continued to highlight common weaknesses in the methodology of IPE studies.[7,10,11,15] Such weaknesses include inadequate detail of what the IPE programme/intervention involved and how it was implemented practically; an over-reliance on outcomes being based primarily on learners assessing their own learning/ behaviour; insufficient validated tools to measure behaviour change connected with IPE and infrequent use of explicit theory to guide the IPE and/or the research methodology (see Box 8.2 for an example of theory within a review methodology). For example, a scoping review of leadership in primary care IPE found that only 9% of the articles stated their theoretical basis, despite the field of leadership being so theoretically rich.[16] O'Carroll et al. state that mixed methods would be most beneficial as purely quantitative can leave questions regarding enablers and barriers, and qualitative often focus on a defined unit and not consider the wider

---

BOX 8.1   THEORY INFORMED IPE RESEARCH[17]

Three universities in the UK developed a common IPE curriculum framework which was deployed across their professional health and care programmes. This involved three strands which ran across the years of each programme and progressed from initial classroom-based teaching on team working and theories to engaging directly with patients in community settings, workshops and simulations. The evaluation of the IPE framework was designed around the Biggs' 3 P Model (which considers the presage, process and product or outputs of students learning), and IPE adapted Kirkpatrick outcome levels. Mixed methods were deployed including validated questionnaires, surveys, focus groups, interviews and workshops.

BOX 8.2   THEORY INFORMED IPE REVIEW[18]

Mertens et al. used a realist review methodology as an interpretative, theory-driven evidence synthesis to understand how and why different outcomes have been observed in a sample of primary studies. To understand the process of workplace learning through collaboration in primary health care, the links between context (C), mechanisms (M) and outcomes (O) were explored. They framed workplace learning in their introduction within sociocultural learning theories and social cognitive learning theories. The analysis of the results according to the CMO principle was then compared to these theories to confirm or adjust insights. Additional learning theories at the individual level were used to understand results that did not match learning as an interactional process.

environment.[5] Reeves et al. suggest though that methods are becoming more robust over time, with increased numbers of quasi-experimental, mixed methods and longitudinal studies.[11]

A common gap across all IPE research is that studies tend to focus on learner-related outcomes and less on changes in individual behaviour, organisational behaviour and changes to care to people and families.[8] In relation to primary care, other research gaps include – the involvement of patients and family carers within the education design and delivery; engaging managers as both learners and/or stakeholders of IPE; the development of leaders and leadership through IPE and team-based processes and outcomes.[6,16,18] Due to the diversity of professions with primary care, and the introduction of new roles such as physician associates and social prescribers, more research needs to be completed regarding the engagement of different professionals. An interesting aspect of this relates to the perception of doctors to IPE. They are in many ways best placed to lead primary care teams towards more integrated care due to their structural influence and traditional role as main decision makers.[16,19,20] However, studies suggest that they are commonly the least positive profession regarding the benefits of IPE.[5] There is also a need to understand how to support other professionals to develop the confidence to take up leadership within collaborative settings.

CONCLUSION

The continued focus on improved collaboration within primary care means there is a pressing need for more research to understand the role of IPE. This should include the most effective educational designs for different contexts and purposes, what is realistic in improved health and well-being of individuals and families, and how IPE can be implemented within challenging organisational and policy contexts. There is no doubt that researching IPE contains additional challenges beyond that within uni-professional settings. It requires researchers to understand the language, traditions and assumptions of other academic disciplines. Translation of IPE findings into practice must speak to more than one set of professional and academic stakeholders (and their host organisations), which again requires the researchers to understand and respond to their differences. And, of course, research teams themselves should ideally be in nature, with all the associated dynamics regarding the successful coordination interdisciplinary of interdisciplinary teams.

Whilst this may initially seem daunting, IPE also provides a unique opportunity for primary care researchers to gain insights from other academic disciplines, and to test out their methods and skills in a new context. Research is about exploring new boundaries of knowledge, and IPE provides a dynamic and important environment to explore.

OPEN ACCESS AND OTHER RESOURCES

Centre for the Advancement of Interprofessional Education: UK-based charity with international outreach whose members (individuals, service users, students and corporate organisations) works together to promote and develop the health and well-being of individuals, families and communities through IPE, collaborative practice and related research facilitating the development of a workforce fit for purpose. Available at: https://www.caipe.org/

O'Carroll V, Owens M, Sy M, et al. Top tips for interprofessional education and collaborative practice research: a guide for students and early career researchers. *J Interprof Care* 2020: 1–6. Available from: https://www.tandfonline.com/doi/full/10.1 080/13561820.2020.1777092

Reeves S, Boet S, Zierler B, Kitto S. Interprofessional education and practice guide no. 3: evaluating interprofessional education. *J Interprof Care* 2015;29(4):305–312. Available from: https://www.tandfonline.com/doi/full/10.3109/13561820. 2014.1003637

University of Michigan Library has developed an Interprofessional Education and Practice Research Guide. This web-based guide pulls together IPE library resources, journals, toolkits and more, in one easy-to-access location. Available at: https://guides.lib. umich.edu/c.php?g=472006&p=6310429

REFERENCES

1. World Health Organization. Framework for action on interprofessional education and collaborative practice. WHO; 2010. Available from: https://apps.who.int/iris/bitstream/handle/10665/70185/WHO_HRH_HPN_10.3_eng.pdf;jsessionid=E48FAA8B3D1DC61B79FF9B1DB501A5A0?sequence=1

2. Samuelson M, Tedeschi P, Aarendonk D, De La Cuesta C, Groenewegen P. Improving inter-professional collaboration in primary care: position paper of the European Forum for Primary Care. *Qual Prim Care* 2012;20(4):303–312.

3. Valentijn PP, Boesveld IC, Van der Klauw DM, et al. Towards a taxonomy for integrated care: a mixed-methods study. *Int J Integr Care* 2015;15(1). DOI:10.5334/ijic.1513.

4. Mangan C, Miller R, Ward C. Knowing me, knowing you. *J Integr Care* 2015;23(2):62–73.

5. O'Carroll V, McSwiggan L, Campbell M. Health and social care professionals' attitudes to interprofessional working and interprofessional education: a literature review. *J Interp Care* 2016;30(1):42–49.

6. Illingworth P, Chelvanayagam S. The benefits of interprofessional education 10 years on. *Br J Nurs* 2017;26(14):813–818.

7. Blue AV, Chesluk BJ, Conforti LN, Holmboe ES. Assessment and evaluation in interprofessional education: exploring the field. *J Allied Health* 2015;44(2):73–82.

8. Reeves S, Fletcher S, Barr H, et al. A BEME systematic review of the effects of interprofessional education: BEME Guide No. 39. *Med Teach* 2016;38(7):656–668.

9. Miller R, Scherpbier N, van Amsterdam L, Guedes V, Pype P. Inter-professional education and primary care: EFPC position paper. *Prim Health Care Res Dev* 2019;20:1–10.

10. Herath C, Zhou Y, Gan Y, Nakandawire N, Gong Y, Lu Z. A comparative study of interprofessional education in global health care: a systematic review. *Medicine* 2017;96(38):1–7.

11. Reeves S, Palaganas J, Zierler B. An updated synthesis of review evidence of interprofessional education. *J. Allied Health* 2017;46(1):56–61.

12. Biggs JB. From theory to practice: a cognitive systems approach. *High Educ Res Dev* 1993;12(1):73–85.

13. Barr H, Koppel I, Reeves S, Hammick M, Freeth DS. *Effective Interprofessional Education: Argument, Assumption and Evidence (Promoting Partnership for Health)*. London: Blackwell; 2005.

14. Parsell G, Bligh J. The development of a questionnaire to assess the readiness of health care students for interprofessional learning (RIPLS). *Med Educ* 1999;33(2):95–100.

15. Gillan C, Lovrics E, Halpern E, Wiljer D, Harnett N. The evaluation of learner outcomes in interprofessional continuing education: a literature review and an analysis of survey instruments. *Med Teach* 2011;33(9):e461–e470.

16. Nieuwboer MS, van der Sande R, van der Marck MA, Olde Rikkert MG, Perry M. Clinical leadership and integrated primary care: a systematic literature review. *Eur J Gen Pract* 2019;25(1):7–18.

17. Anderson E, Smith R, Hammick M. Evaluating an interprofessional education curriculum: a theory-informed approach. *Med Teach* 2016;38(4):385–394.

18. Mertens F, de Groot E, Meijer L, et al. Workplace learning through collaboration in primary healthcare: a BEME realist review of what works, for whom and in what circumstances: BEME guide no. 46. *Med Teach* 2018;40(2):117–134.

19. Grol SM, Molleman GR, Kuijpers A, et al. The role of the general practitioner in multidisciplinary teams: a qualitative study in elderly care. *BMC Fam Pract* 2018;19(1):40.

20. Brewer ML, Flavell HL, Trede F, Smith M. A scoping review to understand "leadership" in interprofessional education and practice. *J Interprof Care* 2016;30(4):408–415.

CHAPTER 9

Research on patient education in primary care

Serap Cifcili

Patient education (PE) is the key element of almost all encounters in clinical practice.[1] More than any other health care workers, primary health care providers should support their patients to adopt a healthy lifestyle for prevention of diseases and to maintain quality of life. In today's medical environment, chronic disease management comprises the bulk of clinical work. Empowering patients to improve their self-management skills is probably the most effective strategy to achieve desired patient outcomes.[2] Therefore, evidence on the effectiveness of PE for a variety of problems in primary care is needed.

'The Research Agenda for General Practice/Family Medicine and Primary Health Care in Europe', developed by the European General Practice Research Network in 2010, emphasises the lack of randomised controlled trials (RCTs) of non-pharmacological interventions, in primary care/general practice.[3] However, in the past decade, research has been published on educating patients in chronical disease self-management skills involving various health workers, mostly nurses. Common topics are management of diabetes, hypertension, cardiac diseases, obesity or weight management, asthma management, chronic pain management and mental health issues.[4-6] Although fewer in number, PE research also has been used in acute diseases.[7] However, in some of these studies, although patients were recruited from primary care settings, the intervention was carried out by an outside health care worker,[8,9] or the settings were community-based specialised health facilities for a specific disease, not a typical primary care clinic in which the providers should deal with a variety of patients with different health problems.[10] In addition, many of them employed complex interventions provided by a team of health care workers.[11] Thus, transferability of the results of these studies to various primary care settings, especially in low- and middle-income countries, might be problematic.[12] In addition, although there are many examples of PE research in primary care setting, there is still a need for well-designed and pragmatic studies transferable to primary care settings in different populations.

WHICH TYPES OF RESEARCH CAN BE USED IN PE?

The best possible research design to evaluate effectiveness of an intervention is to conduct an RCT. However, in RCTs, all the parameters that could possibly affect the trial outcomes are strictly controlled to avoid potential confounders. Thus, many authors suggest that results of RCTs may not always apply to real clinical practice.[12] Primary care settings present additional challenges for RCTs, especially for educational intervention studies. As described in the book *How to Do Primary Care Research*', to provide allocation concealment in primary care setting may not always be possible, thus generally cluster randomisation is preferred.[13] Another issue discussed in the same chapter is the problem of blinding. In educational research, it may be difficult for the researcher to be blind to the allocation groups. However, the person who collects outcome data should be blind to the allocation groups.[13,14]

Nevertheless, a well-designed RCT may be the best way to show effectiveness of a complex educational intervention.[14] An educational RCT example from primary care is presented in Box 9.1.[15]

Quasi-experimental (QE) design is widely used in PE studies. These studies are usually preferred over RCTs due to ethical or practical reasons. An important advantage of QE studies is that their results might be more applicable to the real world. These studies can be used, and widely preferred, to evaluate effectiveness of an educational intervention.[16] Most commonly used QE designs are non-equivalent groups post-test only, non-equivalent groups pre-test post-test and time series.[17] See example in Box 9.2.[18]

An important weakness of both RCTs and QE trials is lack of contextual information or qualitative data such as patients' and providers' experiences. If the aim is to evaluate how a certain education effects the participants, rather than the effectiveness of a given educational intervention, then a qualitative design is needed. Combination of qualitative and quantitative methods (multi-method designs) may answer many challenges in health care research.[19]

Once research type(s) are chosen in concordance with the research question and considering the resources and setting, well-known guidelines of that type(s) of research should be followed. However, certain aspects specifically related to 'education' need to be addressed when conducting patient educational research. Table 9.1 lists these together with sample quotes from a study evaluating the effectiveness of a primary care nurse-delivered

BOX 9.1 EXAMPLE OF A RANDOMISED, SINGLE-BLIND, CONTROLLED PE TRIAL

My first mentorship experience for a dissertation thesis was in 2010. Together with my student, we were interested in a common problem, knee osteoarthritis. In routine practice, we were explaining the benefits of quadriceps-strengthening exercises to these patients, and providing a simple written brochure with drawings along with weight loss advice if needed. However, many patients did not adhere to these exercise instructions. We noticed that if we simply show only one or two exercises to the patients and make them repeat these exercises in our practice right after explanations, and gradually increase exercise intensity, the patients seem to adhere better. Based on this observation and after a thorough literature search, we designed an RCT. With poor human capacity and no funding, we could only use our practice. Since we were unable to recruit many patients from a single centre, our sample size was small. We allocated patients to intervention and control groups with simple 1:1 randomisation. The intervention group received a graded exercise education by demonstration and coaching, and the control group received usual care as described above. Patients in both groups were asked to keep a schematic diary, sign the days when they did the exercises including time and intensity. To avoid bias, both groups received follow-up phone calls and visits. Only the intervention group received an additional visit in which we provided a second-level exercise education. Outcome measures were adherence to exercise which was measured by patient diaries and follow-up phone calls and improvement of functional capacity measured with a commonly used scale.

However, we had to work through several limitations. Firstly, as this was an educational study, neither the primary researcher nor the participants were blinded. To overcome, or at least weaken this limitation, the primary outcome measure (adherence) was assessed by a blinded researcher. Another problem we struggled with that keeping diary and follow-up phone calls created a behavioural change effect in the control group as well. As a result, patients in both groups adhered to recommendations and their functional capacity improved. However, the intervention group improved more than the control group. With a small sample size, single-blind design and short follow-up period results of this study should be evaluated carefully. However, since the study was carried out in a small practice, along with usual daily work, I can argue that our results might easily transferred to many other primary care practices.

educational intervention.[20] These details provide practitioners with the chance to consider whether they can apply the same or similar education methods in their own practice and increase the external validity of the study.

BOX 9.2 EXAMPLE OF A QUASI-EXPERIMENTAL STUDY[18]

The study is designed to evaluate ongoing group medical visits for diabetic patients. These visits combine one-on-one provider visits and group diabetes self-management education. The programme has been evaluated with several RCTs or pilot studies and found to be effective. However, no study evaluated ongoing programmes. Data were extracted from electronic records. A group of patients who had attended at least one practice visit were included in the intervention group, while the control group was extracted from the patients from the same centre who did not participate any of these visits, and were similar to the intervention group in terms of various socio-demographic characteristics. Clinical outcomes such as HbA1C and BMI were evaluated.

The authors chose QE design to evaluate effectiveness of this PE programme as an RCT was not possible, given that the programme was already underway in a large-scale family medicine practice. Although its retrospective and non-randomised design limits its power, by creating a matching control group, the authors tried to minimise confounders. In addition, the study reflects real-life data.

TABLE 9.1 What to address in PE research

Study Characteristics to Be Reported	Example from Study[20]
Setting/characteristics of the primary care centre	'… a primary care centre' (no additional detail)
Method(s) of education (should be in concordance with the aim)	'Structured, individualised, based on goal setting and motivational interviewing (MI)'
Face-to-face or remote	Face-to-face
Media of education (meeting room, physician's/nurse's office, etc.)	Not specified
Timing (duration of every session, if repeated frequency)	Six sessions, 30 minutes each
Group or individual/number of participants in each session	Individual
Qualifications and characteristics of the trainers	'… one trained nurse more than 10 years of experience'
Third parties in the sessions	'… accompanied by a family member, caregiver'
Content of the education sessions	'basic knowledge of diabetes, healthy eating, physical activity, self-monitoring of blood glucose, risk reduction, problem solving, coping skills'

TABLE 9.1 (*Continued*)

Study Characteristics to Be Reported	Example from Study[20]
Patients' participation in the session	Not mentioned, however, MI technique which requires patient participation is used
Additional material	'A brochure containing educational contents, control objectives, and a self-management booklet'
Follow-up sessions	'... educational reinforcements after 12 and 18 months'

In conclusion, primary care providers spend considerable time on PE. Little of the knowledge and expertise gained is disseminated to their primary care peers. Sharing this experience with peers through well-designed studies will enhance primary care practice, and improve the quality of the service provided to the patients.

REFERENCES

1. Svavarsdóttir MH, Sigurðardóttir ÁK, Steinsbekk A. How to become an expert educator: a qualitative study on the view of health professionals with experience in patient education. *BMC Med Educ* 2015;15(1):87. Available from: https://bmcmededuc. biomedcentral.com/articles/10.1186/s12909-015-0370-x

2. Rochfort A, Beirne S, Doran G, et al. Does patient self-management education of primary care professionals improve patient outcomes: a systematic review. *BMC Fam Pract* 2018;19(1):163. Available from: https://bmcfampract.biomedcentral.com/articles/10.1186/s12875-018-0847-x

3. van Royen P, Beyer M, Chevallier P, et al. The research agenda for general practice/family medicine and primary health care in Europe. Part 3. Results: person centred care, comprehensive and holistic approach. *Eur J Gen Pract* 2010;16(2):113–119. Available from: http://www.tandfonline.com/doi/full/10.3109/13814788.2010.481018

4. Correia JC, Lachat S, Lagger G, Chappuis F, Golay A, Beran D. Interventions targeting hypertension and diabetes mellitus at community and primary healthcare level in low- and middle-income countries: a scoping review. *BMC Pub Health* 2019;19(1):1542. Available from: https://bmcpublichealth.biomedcentral.com/articles/10.1186/s12889-019-7842-6

5. Werner EL, Storheim K, Løchting I, Wisløff T, Grotle M. Cognitive patient education for low back pain in primary care. *Spine* 2016;41(6):455–462. Available from: http://journals.lww.com/00007632-201603150-00001

6. Petersen JJ, Hartig J, Paulitsch MA, et al. Classes of depression symptom trajectories in patients with major depression receiving a collaborative care intervention. *PLOS ONE* 2018;13(9):e0202245. Available from: https://dx.plos.org/10.1371/journal.pone.0202245

7. Lemiengre MB, Verbakel JY, Colman R, et al. Reducing inappropriate antibiotic prescribing for children in primary care: a cluster randomised controlled trial of two interventions. *Br J Gen Pract* 2018;68(668):e204–e210. Available from: http://bjgp.org/lookup/doi/10.3399/bjgp18X695033

8. Jolly K, Sidhu MS, Hewitt CA, et al. Self management of patients with mild COPD in primary care: randomised controlled trial. *BMJ* 2018;k2241. Available from: https://www.bmj.com/lookup/doi/10.1136/bmj.k2241

9. Traeger AC, Lee H, Hübscher M, Skinner IW, Moseley GL, Nicholas MK, Henschke N, Refshauge KM, Blyth FM, Main CJ, Hush JM, Lo S, McAuley JH. Effect of Intensive Patient Education vs Placebo Patient Education on Outcomes in Patients With Acute Low Back Pain: A Randomized Clinical Trial. *JAMA Neurol.* 2019 Feb 1;76(2):161–169

10. Chao MT, Hurstak E, Leonoudakis-Watts K, et al. Patient-reported outcomes of an integrative pain management program implemented in a primary care safety net clinic: a quasi-experimental study. *J Gen Intern Med* 2019;34(7):1105–1107. Available from: http://link.springer.com/10.1007/s11606-019-04868-0

11. Wylie-Rosett J, Groisman-Perelstein AE, Diamantis PM, et al. Embedding weight management into safety-net pediatric primary care: randomized controlled trial. *IJBNPA* 2018;15(1):12. Available from: https://ijbnpa.biomedcentral.com/articles/10.1186/s12966-017-0639-z

12. Zuidgeest MGP, Goetz I, Groenwold RHH, Irving E, van Thiel GJMW, Grobbee DE. Series: pragmatic trials and real world evidence: paper 1. Introduction. *J Clin Epi* 2017 Aug;88:7–13. Available from: https://linkinghub.elsevier.com/retrieve/pii/S0895435617305401

13. Bartlett-Esquilant G, Dickinson M, Schuster T. Chapter 21: randomised trials in primary care. In: Goodyear-Smith F, Mash B, eds. *How To Do Primary Care Research.* 1st ed. Boca Raton, FL: CBC Press; 2018. 203–211.

14. Hutchison D, Styles B. *A Guide to Running Randomized Controlled Trials for Educational Researchers.* Slough: National Foundation for Educational Research; 2010:1–7.

15. Tüzün S, Çifçili S, Akman M, Topsakal N, Kalaça S, Cöbek PU. How can we improve adherence to exercise programs in patients with osteoarthritis? A randomized controlled trial. *Turk Geriatri Dergisi* 2012;15(3):513–521.

16. Bärnighausen T, Røttingen J-A, Rockers P, Shemilt I, Tugwell P. Quasi-experimental study designs series—paper 1: introduction: two historical lineages. *J Clin Epi* 2017;89: 4–11. Available from: https://linkinghub.elsevier.com/retrieve/pii/S0895435617307485

17. Gribbons B, Herman J. True and quasi-experimental designs. *PARE* 1996;5(14):1–3.

18. Cunningham AT, Delgado DJ, Jackson JD, et al. Evaluation of an ongoing diabetes group medical visit in a family medicine practice. *J Am Board Fam Med* 2018;31(2): 279–281. Available from: http://www.jabfm.org/lookup/doi/10.3122/jabfm.2018.02.170373

19. Hansen HP, Tjørnhøj-Thomsen T. Meeting the challenges of intervention research in health science: an argument for a multimethod research approach. *Patient* 2016;9(3):193–200. Available from: http://link.springer.com/10.1007/s40271-015-0153-9

20. de la Fuente Coria MC, Cruz-Cobo C, Santi-Cano MJ. Effectiveness of a primary care nurse delivered educational intervention for patients with type 2 diabetes mellitus in promoting metabolic control and compliance with long-term therapeutic targets: randomised controlled trial. *Int J Nurs Stud.* 2020 Jan;101:103417. Available from: https://linkinghub.elsevier.com/retrieve/pii/S002074891930224x

CHAPTER 10

Finding out what is already known: how to develop a literature review

Sophie Park,
Rebecca Rees and
Claire Duddy

WHY DO A LITERATURE REVIEW?

Any research project needs to describe the contribution it makes to existing fields of knowledge. A literature review enables you to learn from relevant texts, progress to become expert in your topic of enquiry and produce new knowledge to address identified gaps. Becoming familiar with existing research and practice helps you understand and describe the ways your contribution fits into, complements or contrasts with existing knowledge. A review is fundamental to the learning process, shaping how you conduct your research. When published, literature reviews often appear discrete and linear. In reality, moving between your own thinking and published texts is integral to ongoing research.

It is easy to assume that your body of literature already exists: it does not and how you create and design it shapes the focus of your review. How you determine which literature is relevant will be unique to your project. It is important to reflexively plan and explicitly describe your approach, but there is no 'right' way to select literature and assess its quality and relevance. Instead, keep asking yourself about the purpose of your review. This helps justify how and why you applied a particular approach and made specific knowledge claims.

This chapter focuses on literature reviews for a research project. Many principles are also relevant to conducting a formal systematic review.[1-3]

WORKING WITH OTHERS

Whilst researchers often conduct informal literature reviews alone, consulting and collaborating with others can be extremely productive. People with different perspectives (e.g. patients, educators or clinical managers) can help identify key concepts and terminology, and highlight gaps and overlooked aspects of a topic. The value of patient and public involvement (PPI) is well-established,[4] and essential to any systematic review proposal; for example, in meta-ethnography,[5,6] realist[7] and configurative reviews.[8,9] Librarians and other information specialists can advise on planning your search and managing the resulting data. Collectively, this provides insight into what is already known, and what it could be useful to know.

DEVELOPING YOUR RESEARCH QUESTION: DECIDING WHAT IS IMPORTANT AND FEASIBLE

Focus first on your research question(s). To help frame these, familiarise yourself with existing literature before embarking on a methodical search. A useful place to start is with academic search engines (e.g. Google Scholar or Microsoft Academic). These are easy to search, and will only find results identified as academic. This approach will not identify a large and unbiased set of relevant literature – see section 'Searching for Relevant Literature' on search sources – but will give a broad understanding of what has been written on your topic.

It may be difficult to know where to start, but start somewhere. Read what others have done and let that shape your own focus and approach. Familiarise yourself with existing knowledge, identify papers of 'key' or 'peripheral' interest and find the 'gap' you want to address. By reading and discussing your topic, you can explore and limit the boundaries of your project, clarifying what is relevant and valuable for you. Common challenges include deciding on the setting, methods, types of learners and dates of interest. Do not try to cover everything in one review. Keep a note of anything you might be interested in to explore in future projects.

The study characteristics (more formally, 'inclusion criteria') you select depend upon the purpose and focus of your review. Randomised controlled trials (RCTs), for example, will help examine intervention effectiveness. Qualitative research and stakeholder experiences are more relevant if exploring how and why something works. No literature review is perfect. All are limited in some way; especially rapid reviews of new innovations. However, these can still contribute to practice and policy, and identify gaps for future research.

After setting some boundaries, consider the range of terms that describe your topic. A librarian can help you with terminology (and synonyms), mapping similarities and differences. For example, the terms 'vocational medical education', 'postgraduate medical education', 'registrar training' and 'medical residency' have commonalities, but differ in the students/trainees, staff and educational possibilities they cover. By clarifying definitions with colleagues, and including appropriate terminology in your search strings, you maximise opportunities for inclusivity, diversity and recognition of globally relevant work. Examine the search terms in the 'methods' sections of published systematic reviews. Many are collected in specialist databases, such as the Cochrane Library, the Campbell Collaboration and the EPPI-Centre and Social Systems Evidence. If you re-use or adapt a published search strategy, remember to cite it.

SEARCHING FOR RELEVANT LITERATURE

Academic literature is collected and indexed in bibliographic databases (Table 10.1). These resources are curated in a systematic and open way by information specialists. ERIC is perhaps the best known educational database, but each database indexes different journals, so choose two or three that complement each other. Librarians can advise on this.

Many bibliographic databases use a standard index of terms ('thesaurus') to label each included reference. Get to know the index terms for your topic in each database as these can be used to retrieve relevant results. A useful shortcut is 'pearl-growing': find a paper which is highly relevant, look at its index terms and build these into your string of search terms.

To create your search strategy, combine search terms (synonyms and index terms) using the Boolean operators 'AND' or 'OR' to build more comprehensive and focussed search strings.

For example, combine sets of search terms using OR:

Set 1, including terms for the setting: 'family medicine' OR 'general practice' OR 'primary care'.
Set 2, including terms for an intervention of interest: 'mobile learning' OR 'online learning' OR 'e-learning'.

Combine these sets using 'AND' (i.e. Set 1 AND Set 2). The output of this search will contain only those papers that use at least one term from each set. Keep records of your search terms for future reviews, and share them with others, who may identify terms you have overlooked.

Identifying relevant literature can be difficult: studies with negative findings are less likely to get published; authors may not use straightforward

TABLE 10.1 Bibliographic databases relevant to health and educational sciences

ERIC (Education Resources Information Center)	Key education journals and reports, dissertations, conference abstracts and teaching materials. https://eric.ed.gov/
British Educational Index (BEI)	British education and training journals, and some international literature. Strengths include education policy and administration.
MEDLINE	US and international biomedical literature Also searchable as part of the PubMed database https://pubmed.ncbi.nlm.nih.gov/
EMBASE	International biomedical and pharmaceutical literature
CINAHL	Nursing, biomedical and allied health professions literature, including journals, books, dissertations, conference proceedings and other material
WHO Global Index Medicus (GIM)	Biomedical and public health literature produced by and within low- and middle-income countries. Comprised of multiple regional databases. http://www.globalindexmedicus.net/
Global Health	International public health literature
Science Citation Index and Social Science Citation Index (via Web of Science)	International science and social science literature from a wide range of disciplines (including health and education)
ASSIA (Applied Social Sciences Index and Abstracts)	English language social science literature from a range of disciplines (including health and education)

titles and promising abstracts may prove to be of peripheral interest. As well as searching databases, review authors often run 'citation searches', by following up citations in relevant papers, and tracking citations forward in time (e.g. using Google Scholar and Web of Science). Remember, recent work may only be available in pre-print, online journals or open peer review platforms. Search outside academic journals for reports from organisations undertaking research, e.g. think tanks, and professional or government body websites (grey literature).[10]

SELECTING, CODING AND GROUPING THE KEY STUDIES

After running searches, you will need to decide which papers to include in your review. Remember the boundaries of your project, and apply the inclusion and exclusion criteria you decided at the start. This is often a two-stage process using titles and abstracts first, then full-text.

You can download and import your search results into reference management software such as Endnote or Mendeley, or dedicated review software such as Covidence, DistillerSR, EPPI-reviewer or Rayyan. These tools enable you to sift through, select and organise references, delete duplicate results and locate, store and annotate electronic copies of documents. A librarian can advise on the best tools for you. If working as a team, some software collaboration tools can record and report the proportion of papers looked at together or individually, and how coding discrepancies were resolved.

You now have a core of papers to consider. For quantitative reviews, look for key data (e.g. absolute risk calculations). For qualitative or mixed methods reviews, familiarise yourself with the papers by asking some questions as you read:

- What is the overall argument?
- What aspect of your topic is covered?
- From what position or perspective (e.g. political, theoretical) is the author writing?
- What claims are made?
- What forms of evidence support these claims?
- How adequate or robust are these claims, within the norms of the methods used?

This process will help you develop and pilot a 'data extraction sheet' to capture and organise key, relevant characteristics of the included studies. You will need to evaluate included papers in a way that suits your overall approach. This might involve informal discussion of relevance and limitations, or using formal quality assessment tools (e.g. CASP Checklists, Cochrane Risk of Bias tool).[11,12]

To decide what findings and contextual information to take from a study, think about what is relevant for your review and purpose. You can simply map or describe the content of each paper. Additionally, you can examine the relationships between papers and various findings. This process enables you both to describe what knowledge exists, and transform available knowledge to produce new insights ('building a jigsaw'). A combination of deductive and inductive analysis can be used. Deductive analysis involves looking for a predefined set of questions or categories within the data. These are likely to have been developed and agreed at the outset, perhaps in collaboration with stakeholders. Inductive analysis involves examining the available data 'bottom up', maximising curiosity about unanticipated or unexpected relevant findings.

Analysis can be time-consuming. It often requires multiple readings of documents to gain familiarity; re-visiting sections after further reading and clarifying and confirming contextual meaning and relevance. A useful approach is to make distinct initial 'data gathering' (extracting, e.g. verbatim quotes from papers in italics, or quantitative data such as effect sizes) from subsequent analysis or 'interpretation' of the extracted data. Interpretation shapes the whole process, from initial selection of 'relevant' data, to the formation (and potential subsequent conflation or separation) of the analytical categories used. There is no 'right' or 'wrong' process: every method has its strengths and limitations. However, by documenting your approach, the reader can understand and critique how and why particular decisions were made.

DISSEMINATING YOUR FINDINGS

How you describe and summarise your review will be shaped by the intended audience and publication constraints. A number of different stories may emerge from the combined texts. You need to consider how to relate that range of possibilities to your research or project goals at that point in time. A literature review may focus on both your topic and methods of interest, enabling readers to understand why and how you have conducted your research in a particular way. You can draw upon existing literature to discuss how your work relates to and contributes to what is already 'known'.

When published, literature reviews tend to appear linear and simple. Doing a literature review, however, involves reading and writing throughout the research process and, can feel unwieldy and at times over-whelming. The word 'review' suggests a passive activity: showing, summarising, collecting. This positions the researcher as an observer of others' work. In reality, doing a literature review is a creative, active and often exhausting process. Used well, it is an opportunity for you to use and evaluate the work of others in producing a place for your own work.

REFERENCES

1. Gough D, Oliver S, Thomas J. *An Introduction to Systematic Reviews.* 2nd ed. Los Angeles: Sage; 2017:331.
2. Booth A, Sutton A, Papaioannou D. *Systematic Approaches to a Successful Literature Review.* 2nd ed. Los Angeles: Sage; 2016:326.
3. Sandelowski M, Barroso J. *Handbook for Synthesizing Qualitative Research.* New York: Springer Publishing. 2006. Pp312.
4. INVOLVE. Available from: https://www.invo.org.uk

5. France EF, Cunningham M, Ring N, et al. Improving reporting of meta-ethnography: the eMERGe reporting guidance. *BMC Med Res Methodol* 2019;19(1):25.
6. Park S, Khan N, Stevenson F, Malpass A. Patient and public involvement (PPI) in evidence synthesis: how the PatMed study approached embedding audience responses into the expression of a meta-ethnography. *BMC Med Res Methodol* 2020;20(1):29.
7. Abrams R, Park S, Wong G, et al. Lost in reviews: looking for the involvement of stakeholders, patients, public and other non-researcher contributors in realist reviews. *Res Synth Methods* 2020;1–9. doi:10.1002/jrsm.1459
8. Rees R, Oliver S. Stakeholder involvement. In: Gough D, Oliver S, Thomas J, eds. *Introduction to Systematic Reviews*. London: Sage; 2017.
9. Oliver K, Rees R, Brady L, Kavanagh J, Oliver S, Thomas J. Broadening public participation in systematic reviews: a case example involving young people in two configurative reviews. *Res Synth Methods* 2015;6(2):206–217.
10. AMEE Links and Resources. The Association for Medical Education in Europe. 2020. Available from: https://amee.org/links-and-resources
11. CASP Checklists. Available from: https://casp-uk.net/casp-tools-checklists/ (Assessed 23 October 2020).
12. Cochrane Risk of Bias tool. Available from https://methods.cochrane.org/bias/resources/rob-2-revised-cochrane-risk-bias-tool-randomized-trials (Accessed 23 October 2020).

CHAPTER 11

Choosing your topic and defining your research question

Helen Reid and Jenny Johnston

INTRODUCTION

This chapter aims to support novice researchers in constructing appropriate research questions in primary care education. The focus is on empirical research, starting with considerations around the research topic, then moving on to defining and refining research questions.

PROBLEMATISING WORK CONTEXTS

Finding an appropriate area to research may seem baffling to begin with, given the overwhelming breadth of available material. It is often helpful for researchers to start by thinking about their own work contexts; for example, by reflecting on what seems interesting, challenging or just plain difficult. The needs of patients, students, health care professionals and other stakeholders should be considered, as they are experienced in everyday working life. How might people benefit, or systems change, as a result of an educational study? This all-important 'so what' question should be addressed at the earliest possible stage. Ultimately, research in primary care education is about driving social change in health care. Does researching this topic matter? Who stands to benefit from it? Will other people care, beyond the local context?

Once a broad topic has been determined, consideration must be given to identifying key stakeholders. Novice researchers and those undertaking postgraduate degrees will often join an existing stream of research work. It is important at the outset to establish whether there is complete freedom, or (more usually) what constraints exist in terms of time, resources, funding or commitment to contribute to an existing research project or programme. This helps to locate the problem within various contexts. Finding a way for research to 'join' an existing conversation or debate means a ready-made audience, but it is also possible to design entirely new research questions and streams. This is particularly relevant in settings where there may not be an established history of primary care education research, or where rapid change is happening. The coronavirus pandemic is a key example of a paradigm shift, creating an urgent need for adaptations to learning and teaching, with a consequent need for high-quality educational research (Box 11.1).

UNDERSTANDING SCALE AND IMPACT

For any given topic, there will be a plethora of possible research questions. Often it is choosing the most relevant, which is the challenge. Setting the right scale is vital. It is easy to make questions too broad (unanswerable within research constraints) or too narrow (of limited relevance and impact). Note, however, that questions which start out 'local and particular' can often be developed into having broader relevance.

Lingard's popular Problem-Gap-Hook framework[1] is one way to address the issue of scale when designing research questions. Articulating the context is followed by defining the research need, in terms of new knowledge or practice, and finally the 'hook' is considered; that is, how the final research product might spark interest or impact others. This is a pragmatic way to reduce unwieldy ideas into concise, useful questions without diluting impact.

BOX 11.1 POTENTIAL STAKEHOLDERS IN PRIMARY CARE EDUCATION RESEARCH

- Students and educators across health care disciplines
- Practising clinicians
- Patients and the public
- Policymakers
- Guideline developers
- Primary care commissioning groups
- Professional organisations/collaborations
- Universities
- Health care systems
- Governments

UNITS OF ANALYSIS

Primary care education research may encompass any area of working life where learning and development take place. Thus, while formal educational contexts, such as university primary care modules and postgraduate training schemes, are familiar subjects, research can also extend into diverse aspects of informal workplace (on the job) learning.

The subject of the research question is known as the unit of analysis. This may range from a single consultation or computer entry to individuals, teams, organisations, programmes of study or entire health care systems.

METHODOLOGICAL CONSIDERATIONS

Research questions need to be developed concurrently with choosing an appropriate methodology (overall research approach) and methods (the practical 'tools' of the research). It is an essential part of rigour that these are aligned and congruent with one other, meaning they share underlying assumptions about what they are setting out to achieve.[2]

For example, qualitative research is often exploratory, using 'how' or 'why' questions. These may be best answered using qualitative methodologies such as thematic analysis, grounded theory, phenomenology or discourse analysis (Chapter 19). The practical methods associated might include interviews, focus groups, participant observation or documentary analysis. Quantitative research, on the other hand, is commonly explanatory, using 'what' or 'how much' questions. Methods might include measurements, questionnaires or randomised controlled trials, followed by statistical analysis (Chapter 15). It is also possible to set two related research questions in a mixed methods study, for example, combining a quantitative questionnaire with follow-up qualitative interviews. This approach is gaining in popularity (see Chapter 25).[3]

DRAWING IT ALL TOGETHER

After so much thinking, it is time to start drawing everything together. Discussion is helpful at this refining stage. Within medical schools, undergraduate researchers are well placed to collaborate within their universities with experienced primary care researchers and harness the support of behavioural scientists (Chapter 3). Postgraduate researchers will have a supervisory team, and may have a community of practice from which to draw support. For researchers in clinical practice, seeking mentorship, peer support and stakeholder input is equally valuable.

When wording a final research question, it may be helpful to draw on a familiar tool such as PICO (patient, intervention, control/comparison, outcome),[4] commonly used in biomedical research, to which many new primary care education researchers will have been exposed (Chapter 26). A similar tool, SPIDER (Sample, Phenomenon of Interest, Design, Evaluation, Research type) can be used for qualitative questions.[5]

CONCLUSION

A good research question, one that matters and has the potential to engender a positive change, is worth taking time to develop. In the authors' experience, most go through many iterations. Indeed, in some educational research, ongoing iteration between question and data continues in parallel, and the question may be continually refined as the research progresses. Time spent thinking around your topic and developing your research question is time well spent, if your goal is rigorous and meaningful research.

REFERENCES

1. Lingard L. Joining a conversation: the problem/gap/hook heuristic. *Perspect Med Educ* 2015;4:252–253.
2. Carter SM, Little M. Justifying knowledge, justifying method, taking action: epistemologies, methodologies, and methods in qualitative research. *Qual Health Res* 2007;17(10):1316–1328.
3. Johnson RB, Onwuegbuzie AJ. Mixed methods research: a research paradigm whose time has come. *Educ Res* 2004;33(7):14–26.
4. Schard C, Adams MB, Owens T, Keitz S, Fontelo P. Utilization of the PICO framework to improve searching PubMed for clinical questions. *BMC Med Inform Decis Mak* 2007;7(1):16.
5. Cooke A, Smith D, Booth A. Beyond PICO: the SPIDER tool for qualitative evidence synthesis. *Qual Health Res* 2012;22(10):1435–1443.

CHAPTER 12

Choosing your methodology to answer your question

Arzu Uzuner

INTRODUCTION

Educational research is a component of undergraduate education, vocational training and of continuing professional development in primary care. The research planning process begins with a research question, and continues with choosing an appropriate method that enables the researcher to answer this question.

Research methods are basically defined as quantitative, qualitative or mixed types, and described by using different characteristics of the study such as data collection techniques (observational/documentation/review), data characteristics (primary data/secondary data), aim (basic/descriptive/experimental/analytic), timing of data collection (instantaneous/cross-sectional/longitudinal/prospective/retrospective), number of participant or observation unit (mono-participant/multi-participant), experiment-measure conditions (intergroup/ingroup-mixed design) and manipulation/intervention status (experimental/non-experimental).[1-4]

Choosing the most appropriate research method depends on many different criteria: the nature of the question and existing data, the facilities that enable the researcher to undertake the study, the barriers that limit its realisation and finally the competencies of the researcher (Table 12.1).[2,5,6]

Primary care researchers work within three main research areas: teaching, organisation and clinical service delivery. Some teaching and educational research topics are listed below:

- Evaluation of primary care education outcomes in undergraduate, specialty/vocational training, continuing professional development
- Need assessment for new competencies for health care providers
- New educational methods, new technologies and new tendencies in education
- Use and effectiveness of online education
- Effectiveness of computer-based examinations versus conventional methods
- Impacts of teaching involvement on clinical teachers, their colleagues and patients[7-9]
- Impact of teaching and learning on teachers and learners, and their professional life[7]
- Perceptions, preferences, challenges of the primary care workers[7,10]

TOPICS, QUESTIONS AND METHODS

Here are some examples of how to find appropriate research method for specific research questions.

Suppose that you are planning a course or a training programme for primary health care providers. This will include an intervention to develop their knowledge and professional skills. Some of the questions to be answered are:

- How effective would the course/programme be?
- How much will the training contribute to the knowledge or competencies of the trainees in the long term?
- What content will be appropriate for the participants?
- Are the trainers competent enough to transfer the knowledge?

Each question could be a proposal for a research plan, and the methodology depends mainly on the aim and definition of the question, as well as the other criterion listed in Table 12.1. The effectiveness of the training will be usually shown by the statistically significant difference in the knowledge of the participants before and after training. For this purpose, you can plan pre- and post-tests with multiple-choice, true/false, or fill-in-the-blanks type questions. Attitudinal and behavioural changes need more observation-based methods such as using checklists and observing the participant's performance on the job or using item-based questions for behaviour or case-based questions for the attitude. All this information can be converted into numbers, which means that a quantitative research methodology will be appropriate for this purpose.

TABLE 12.1 Criteria for choosing the appropriate research methodology

Criteria	Definition
Type of question	Educational, clinic-laboratory-community based/epidemiological
Aim of question	Description or causality
Existing data	Information that already exists Unknown parts of the topic that remain to be enlightened No data
Presence of sociocultural, psychological challenges	Sociocultural characteristics, barriers, Grey zone topics or sensitive issues such as child abuse or violence
Practical considerations	Availability of the resources such as economic or skilled manpower Need for laboratory means Presence and number of participants and their willingness for participation Availability and attainability of data Procedure to get permission from institutions Environmental conditions Timeframe/schedule for the study
Researcher characteristics	Capability and competency Experience in certain methods Tendency to certain research types Collaboration and communication competencies with other researchers

In order to develop the course you might need to use different research methods, according to your question:

- Which content would be appropriate for the participants? – Descriptive.
- What is the competency level of the trainers who will run the course? – Cross-sectional.
- How much progress the training would create in the knowledge or the competencies of the trainees in the long term? – Prospective.

All these questions are related to observational studies, where the researcher is not intending to make any intervention. However, the question of how effective will the course/programme be? can only be answered by an intervention study. All these examples given until now require quantitative methods.[11,12]

Sometimes analysis can be done retrospectively, such as a study examining the use of theatre in a medical curriculum.[13] In this case, an educational method was evaluated retrospectively using the yearly score of the students and their quantitative and qualitative feedback.

An intervention study could explore the effectiveness of online education or computer-based examinations versus conventional methods. Randomised controlled studies are the best methods to compare and show statistical significance of effectiveness. Intervention studies use experimental methods, performed in an environment where variables can be controlled and manipulated to investigate cause-and-effect relationships.[1,2] A study examining the consistency between clinical and preclinical observers in the formation of medical students' history taking skills used a causal comparative survey model.[14]

The evaluation of an education/training programme which includes many educational activities can be challenging. In this case, assessment tools such as student logbook, formative and/or summative tests or essays and on-the-job observation of the students for clinical competencies by mini-clinical exams or objective structured clinical examinations can be helpful. You may want to evaluate the whole programme retrospectively. In this case, you may design a descriptive, retrospective, quantitative survey and a qualitative inquiry simultaneously. A study of a three-year mandatory student research programme in an undergraduate medical curriculum used a mixed method approach to evaluate this longitudinal, interdisciplinary programme.[15] The outcomes were the number of student projects presented in medical congresses and published in medical journals, and student, graduate and mentor feedback. The latter included qualitative positive and negative feedback.

Some research questions might require only qualitative methodologies to be answered. You may want to explore the perceptions or feelings of a working team, their career choice, the reasons behind their choices. Two examples are a study looking at the influence on London general practitioners of teaching undergraduates,[8] and students' perceptions of advantages and disadvantages of community-based and hospital-based teaching.[10] Qualitative methodology that uses mainly verbal data with an interpretative, subjective approach helps researchers to understand thoughts, concepts or experiences of the participants. Grey zone topics or sensitive issues are best studied qualitatively. Data are collected from a purposely selected sample of participants via structured, semi-structured, unstructured interviews and focus groups. Case studies, discourse analysis, participant observations and literature reviews can be used.[1,4,16]

Research questions about the evaluation of interdisciplinary cooperation and coordination, quality/standards/accreditation or the impact of learning on the learners may need mixed methodology. A study of whether teaching during a general practice consultation affected patient care conducted semi-structured interviews with patients and then questionnaire constructed and distributed to many patients to gather their views.[9] A mixed methods study may begin with a qualitative part where the background data is collected by interviews and documents and their analysis; continue by a quantitative part to be tested in general population or begins with a quantitative part and continue with qualitative part, or both methods used concurrently.[16–19] If there are sufficient existing data, a quantitative-only design may be used, such as in a study of residents' views about family medicine specialty education in Turkey, where the survey questions were drawn from published literature.[20]

In summary, to choose the appropriate method, the researcher should consider many factors, such as existing data, practical availabilities and challenges and tailor the methodology, specifically according to the aim of the question.

REFERENCES

1. Büyüköztürk Ş, Kılıç Çakmak E, Akgün ÖE, Karadeniz Ş, Demirel F. *Scientific Research Methods in Education.* 26th ed. Ankara: Pegem Akademi; 2019: 12. doi:10.14527/9789944919289.
2. Köse E. Scientific research models. In: Kıncal YR, ed. *Scientific Research Methods.* 5th ed. Ankara: Nobel Publishing House; 2017: 99–123.
3. Cohen L, Manion L, Morrison K. *Research Methods in Education.* 6th ed. New York: Taylor & Francis e-Library; 2007.
4. Lodico MG, Spaulding DT, Voegtle KH. *Methods in Educational Research. From Theory to Practice.* 1st ed. San Francisco: Jossey Bass; 2006.
5. Opoku A, Ahmed V, Akotia J. Choosing an appropriate research methodology and method. In: Ahmed V, Opoku A, Aziz Z, eds. *Research Methodology in the Built environment. A Selection of Case Studies.* 1st ed. London: Routledge; 2016: 32–48. doi:10.4324/9781315725529
6. Naude C, Young T. How to search and critically appraise the literature. In: Goodyear-Smith F, Mash B, eds. *How To Do Primary Care Research.* Boca Raton, FL: CRC Press, Taylor & Francis Group; 2019: 138.
7. Park S, Rosenthal J, Harding A. Educational research in primary care: addressing the challenges through creation of a special interest group and a doctoral student Network. *Prim Health Care Res Dev* 2012;13:98–100. doi:10.1017/S146342361100065X
8. Hartley S, Macfarlane F, Gantley M, Murray E. Influence on general practitioners of teaching undergraduates: qualitative study of London general practitioner teachers. *BMJ* 1999;319:1168–1171.
9. O'Flynn N, Spencer J, Jones R. Does teaching during a general practice consultation affect patient care? *Br J Gen Pract* 1999;49:7–9.
10. O'Sullivan M, Martin J, Murray E. Students' perceptions of the relative advantages and disadvantages of community-based and hospital-based teaching: a qualitative study. *Med Educ* 2000;34:648–655.
11. Schuster T. How to conduct observational studies. In: Goodyear-Smith F, Mash B, eds. *How To Do Primary Care Research.* Boca Raton, FL: CRC Press, Taylor & Francis Group; 2019: 195–202.

12. Thiese MS. Observational and interventional study design types; an overview. *Biochem Med* 2014;24(2):199–210. doi:10.11613/BM.2014.022

13. Unalan P, Uzuner A, Çifçili S, Akman M, Hancıoğlu S, Thulesius HO. Using theatre in education in a traditional lecture oriented medical curriculum. *BMC Med Educ* 2009;9(73). doi:10.1186/1472-6920-9-73.

14. Akman M, Cifcili S, Unalan PC, Uzuner A, Kaya CA. Evaluation of the consistency between clinical and preclinical observers in the formation of the history taking skills of fourth year medical students of Marmara University. *Turkiye Klinikleri J Med Sci* 2011;31(4):845–852. doi:10.5336/medsci.2009-14923.

15. Akman M, Unalan PC, Kalaca S, Kaya CA, Cifcili S, Uzuner A. A three-year mandatory student research program in an undergraduate medical curriculum in Turkey. *Kuwait Med J* 2010;42(3):205–210.

16. Choy LT. The strengths and weaknesses of research methodology: comparison and complimentary between qualitative and quantitative approaches. *ISOR J Humanit Soc Sci* 2014;19(4):99–104. doi:10.9790/0837-194399104

17. Fetters MD, Curry LA, Creswell JW. Achieving integration in mixed methods designs-principles and practices. *Health Serv Res* 2013;48(6 Pt 2):2134–2156. doi:10.1111/1475-6773.12117

18. Guetterman TC, Fetters MD, Creswell JW. Integrating quantitative and qualitative results in health science mixed methods research through joint displays. *Ann Fam Med* 2015;13:554–561. doi:10.1370/afm.1865

19. Halcomb E. Combining qualitative and quantitative methods. In: Goodyear-Smith F, Mash B, eds. *How To Do Primary Care Research*. Boca Raton, FL: CRC Press, Taylor & Francis Group; 2019:39–46.

20. Uzuner A, Topsever P, Unluoglu I, et al. Residents' views about family medicine specialty education in Turkey. *BMC Med Educ* 2010;10:29.

CHAPTER 13

Ethical issues for primary care educational research

Tim Dare

INTRODUCTION

Primary care educational research is subject to the ethical requirements and principles that govern research and evaluation in general. In addition, the educational and primary care contexts generate specific concerns, including some that are distinctive of educational research and some that are particular to primary care educational research.

RESEARCH ETHICS AT THE BROADEST LEVEL

It is worth emphasising at the outset that 'research ethics' should not be regarded as primarily directed at 'unethical' researchers. Even 'good' researchers may fail to see potential conflicts or give insufficient weight or consideration to the competing interests of participants when under pressure to produce research or simply filled with enthusiasm for a research project. Research ethics is primarily concerned to help good, well-intentioned researchers avoid such errors and missteps and to produce valuable research, ethically.

It is beyond the scope of this chapter to rehearse in detail the ethical requirements and principles pertaining to research broadly considered. For now, it will do to emphasise the following.

First, researchers must never forget that participants are more than 'mere research material'. We all use things to achieve our goals but there are obvious differences between the things we use that are inanimate objects (my computer, my pen), and those that are people. People have goals, plans, loves, fears, aspirations, and so on. It is these capacities that distinguish them from 'mere objects or material' and make them moral agents. The point is most famously stated by Kant: 'Act so that you treat humanity, whether in your own person or in that of another, always as an end and never as a means only'.[1] When we 'use' people to achieve our goals, we must recognise that status.

Second, whatever harms or burdens research causes or places on participants must be outweighed by anticipated benefits. Particular care to avoid or mitigate potential harm is required when research addresses topics that are 'sensitive' in the sense that they deal with vulnerable participants, or behaviour that is intimate, discreditable, stigmatising or incriminating.[2] Note that benefits need not always accrue to research participants themselves. They may fall to future students or patients, or to larger communities in the form, perhaps, of advances in knowledge. In educational contexts, in particular benefits may be indirect, consisting of the improved expertise of trainee researchers. Such research may be legitimate, although it is unlikely to justify very significant burdens on research participants. Research that will not produce any benefit – perhaps because there is no genuine question to be answered, or because a project is methodologically flawed – will, however, quite probably be unethical, since there will be nothing to outweigh any burdens borne by participants.

CONSENT

Informed consent is fundamental to ethical research. It is not a purely formal or procedural matter – it is not about the signature on the form – and nor is it a discrete one-time event: it should be ongoing and available for review throughout the research process.[3] Ethically, the need for informed consent flows from the foundational obligation to treat others with respect. As remarked, we must recognise the status of participants as moral agents. The most obvious way to do that is to ensure that they have exercised their capacities as moral agents to choose whether to be involved in our projects. That choice – their consent – must be genuine and informed.

This requires the provision of full information before participants consent. Care should be taken to provide information in a form appropriate to participants: if participants in primary care educational research are senior medical students, information might appropriately include technical medical terms with which they can be expected to be familiar; if they are lay-people, the information should be less technical. It may be tempting to provide vast quantities of information, but very long information sheets are unlikely to be read and processed.

Full information may lead participants to modify their behaviour in ways which undermine legitimate research. Researchers must obtain independent assessment and approval before proceeding with such research: they must not act on their own assessment since their interest in the research may lead even good researchers to overvalue the research and to give insufficient weight to the interests of participants. Approval in such cases will depend upon showing that the research is important and poses minimal risk to participants, and that it could not be carried out if participants were fully informed. Usually, participants must be provided with full information as soon as possible.

As remarked, consent must be freely given. Participants may lack a genuine choice if some feature of their relationship with the researcher makes it difficult for them to decline. This threat to the free consent may be present in a wide range of research contexts. Educational researchers should be especially careful when engaging students as participants: students may be reluctant to say no to their teachers or to fellow students. Ideally, participants should not be the students of the researcher. Where they are, care must be taken to ensure that there is no element of coercion, including anything approaching a requirement to participate in order to obtain a qualification or grade. If primary care educational research involves participants who are patients, additional precautions may need to be taken to ensure that consent is freely given: patients may be especially reluctant to disappoint those they perceive themselves to be dependent upon for medical care. More generally, care should always be taken to clearly distinguish the multiple roles and relations which researchers and participants may occupy and not to disregard the duties of primary roles, such as that of educator.

CONFIDENTIALITY, PRIVACY AND ANONYMITY

It is useful to begin discussion of confidentiality, privacy and anonymity by thinking about why preserving agents' control of information about them may be important.

Some reasons tie to basic concerns about harms and benefits. Information given to researchers (about a participant's experiences as a student or patient, for instance) may be used to their detriment, or, equally important, they may reasonably fear that it could be (especially, but not only, when research addresses sensitive topics, in the sense described above). We guard against some of these dangers by ensuring confidentiality (that researchers will disclose information without participant consent) and/or anonymity (that participants are not identifiable).

Respecting participants' interests in controlling information may also flow from more direct interests. It has been suggested that we control access to information about us to create different relationships, with different levels of intimacy: my wife knows almost everything about me; my children and friends, fewer and different things; the stranger on the train almost nothing. Others have argued that privacy allows us to 'try out' different public personas quietly and safely, behind the scenes, before deciding what to take onto the public stage.[4]

These sorts of concerns give us ethical reasons to respect participants' interests in privacy, reasons which are in many jurisdictions supplemented by privacy regulations. They also give us reasons to ensure that information provided by participants is used only with, and consist with, participant consent: it is their information.

Where possible, participants should be able to revoke consent and withdraw from research, taking their information with them. If there are limits to their ability to do so – perhaps because their information has been anonymised and/or aggregated with other information, or because it has already prompted other contributions (so that it cannot be withdrawn without rendering those responses meaningless), those limits should be explained clearly in the information given to participants at the outset.

Focus groups raise other issues for confidentiality and anonymity. While participants should be usually be advised that information given by fellow participants should not be disclosed outside the focus groups, researchers should make clear that they cannot guarantee compliance with such instructions. Researchers have less control over the information given in such contexts than they do over information that can secure on a password-protected computer.

Other limits to anonymity should also made clear where appropriate: even if researchers remove identifying information from reports, given enough information about a research population readers may be able to identify participants. Such identification should be made as difficult as possible; where it cannot be guaranteed, participants should be made aware of the risk and consent to taking it on.[5]

ETHICS AND RESEARCH BEYOND THE MEDICAL MODEL

Many of the central notions of 'research ethics' have emerged from medical research and, in particular, from the research paradigm which assumes that 'random controlled trials' are the gold standard. However, a good deal of primary care educational research is likely to fall outside that narrow paradigm. Much will be qualitative, and in some research design may emerge from iterative engagement with participants, preventing the detailed up-front specification of the project and the role of study participants taken for granted by standard principles of research ethics.[6]

This chapter cannot address all of the specific ethical issues generated by these common forms of educational research. Nevertheless, while the classic principles of research ethics may not apply straightforwardly to such activities, it is nonetheless crucial that they are likely to deliver a balance of benefits over harms and that participants are treated with respect. It may be especially important in projects which grant research-inexperienced participants a role in research design to ensure that they appreciate the potential burdens of participation, including an estimate of the time that will be required, and the possibility that motivating benefits may not be realised.

ETHICAL DILEMMAS AND HARD CASES

The term 'ethical dilemma' is over-used. Strictly speaking an ethical *dilemma* arises when all the options available to an agent are ethically problematic. Fortunately, genuine ethical dilemmas are rare, but there is a tendency to describe almost any ethically demanding situation as a dilemma and such cases are far more common.[7]

We have touched on some already. The provision of full information may undermine research goals; researchers may occupy multiple roles, generating conflicting obligations and preferences. Specific examples seem likely to occur in primary care educational contexts (teachers and students, caregivers and patients), but concerns about the potential significance of relationships between researchers and participants are much broader. An imbalance of power which places participants at a disadvantage with respect to researchers may arise for many reasons beyond those captured by specific relationships.

There are other examples. Research results may suggest that a researcher's colleague not competent or is acting improperly, though the research did not contemplate such a conclusion; a researcher may realise that their results could be used to support problematic policy or administrative decisions, or be misrepresented by interests antithetical to the participants; participants may be allocated to an intervention that a researcher believes will not serve them well.

It is not possible to provide a full list of potentially 'ethically demanding cases', nor to specify hard-and-fast rules for dealing with them. Researchers, especially those who occupy dual roles with participants, as is common in educational and primary care educational research, should proceed with caution, remembering that their primary role and duties as educator are likely to take priority over those as researcher. They should be careful to treat participants with respect, avoid abuse of power and appreciate that their priorities and perspectives may not be shared by participants. They should welcome independent ethical review, seeing it as an opportunity to help them produce good, ethical research.

REFERENCES

1. Kant I. *Foundations of the Metaphysic of Morals*, Vol. 47. Lewis White Beck. Indianapolis: Bobbs-Merril; 1959: 429.
2. Renzetti C, Lee R. Researching sensitive topics. *ICRVAW Faculty Book Gallery 14*, Sage Publications: Newbury Park, USA. 1993.
3. Miller T, Bell L. Consenting to what? Issues of access, gate-keeping and 'informed' consent. In: Miller T, Birch M, Mauthner M, Jessop J, eds. *Ethics in Qualitative Research*. London: SAGE Publications; 2012: 61–75. doi:10.4135/9781473913912

4. Schoeman, F. Privacy: philosophical dimensions. *Am Philos Q* 1984;21(3):199–213.
5. BERA. *Ethical Guidelines for Educational Research.* 4th ed. London; 2018: 40–46. Available from: www.bera.ac.uk/researchers-resources/publications/ethical-guidelines-for-educational-research-2018 (Accessed 16 October 2018).
6. Manzo L, Brightbill N. Toward a participatory ethics'. In: Kindon S, Pain R, Kesby M, eds. *Participatory Action Research Approaches and Methods: Connecting People, Participation and Place*007. Routledge: London, UK 59–66.
7. Burgess R. Ethics and educational research: an introduction. In: Burgess R, ed. *The Ethics of Educational Research.* New York: Falmer Press; 1989.

CHAPTER 14

Validity and reliability in primary care educational research

Wichuda Jiraporncharoen, Chaisiri Angkurawaranon and Mehmet Akman

INTRODUCTION

As in all research, validity and reliability lie at the heart of conducting educational research in primary care. In short, validity refers to how accurately researchers can capture what they intended to measure and how 'truthful' the research results are. Reliability refers to whether the research results can be reproduced and remain consistent given similar methodology.[1] Research results need to be valid and reliable so that findings have their intended impact.

WHAT IS VALIDITY?

In essence, validity refers to how the research measures what it purports to measure. It is usually categorised into internal and external validity. Internal validity refers to how the explanation of a particular event or issue can actually be sustained by the data. The findings must describe accurately the phenomena being researched. External validity is the degree to which the results can be generalised to the wider population, cases or situation. The issue of internal and external validity may differ between quantitative and qualitative research.[1,2]

VALIDITY IN QUANTITATIVE RESEARCH

In quantitative research, validity concerns a specific measurement in a specific situation with a specific group of individuals. Internal validity can be broken down into three major categories: content, criterion-related and construct validity.[1]

- *Content validity* is determined by a review of the assessment instrument and the extent to which it measures what it is intended to measure. The instrument must show that it fairly and comprehensively covers the domain or items that it is purposed to cover. This may affect respondents' motivation to complete a questionnaire and also the time needed to be allocated for it. To establish content validity, the measurement team needs experts to examine the objective and the item of the test.
- *Criterion-related validity* refers to a comparison of the test score against a known criterion of the expected performance. It can tell how the new test is concurrent to the standard test and predict performance in a future situation.[3]
- *Construct validity* refers to a collection of indirect information that the assessment instrument measures what it purports to measure. The operationalised form of a construct is used to clarify the meaning when we use this construct. The researchers need to be assured that their construction of a particular issue agrees with other constructions of the same underlying issue, by referencing the relevant literature.

For external validity, generalisability is interpreted as comparability and transferability. Researchers should make it possible to assess the typicality of a situation, the participants and setting, and indicate how data might translate into different settings and cultures.

VALIDITY IN QUALITATIVE RESEARCH

Qualitative research may require a different framework when assessing for internal validity. It can be broken down into five major categories[2]:

- *Descriptive validity*: The factual accuracy of the account, that it is not made up, selective or distorted – what actually happened.
- *Interpretive validity*: The ability of research to capture the meaning, interpretations, terms, intentions that situations or events have for participants in their terms – what it means to the researched person or group.
- *Theoretical validity*: The theoretical constructions the researchers bring to the research.

- *Generalisability*: The view that the theory generated may be useful in understanding other similar situations.
- *Evaluation validity*: An evaluative, judgemental application of that which is being researched, rather than a descriptive, explanatory framework.

The issue of external validity in qualitative research usually focuses on the fact that it is often aimed at understanding a particular phenomenon which can be context-specific. Researchers should provide clear detailed and in-depth description so that others can decide the extent to which finding from one piece of the research can be generalisable.

WHAT IS RELIABILITY?

Reliable research must be repeatable. This means that when it carried out on a similar group of respondents in a similar context (however defined), then similar results would be found. Similar to the validity, issues relating to reliability also depend on the type of research.

RELIABILITY IN QUANTITATIVE RESEARCH

Reliability in quantitative research is essentially a synonym for dependability, consistency and replicability over time, over instruments and over groups of respondents. It is concerned with precision and accuracy. There are three principal types: stability, equivalence and internal consistency.[2]

- *Reliability as stability* is a measure of consistency over time and over similar samples. A reliable instrument for a piece of research will yield similar data from similar respondents over time. If a test and then a retest were undertaken within an appropriate time span, then similar results would be obtained. An appropriate time scale between the test and retest can be considered by two factors. Firstly, the time period is not advised to be too long, because situational factors may change, or not too short, because the participants might recall the first test. Secondly, participants may be interested in the context and may have developed a deeper understanding of the subject between the test and the retest dates. Correlation coefficients can be calculated for the reliability of pre-tests and post-tests.
- *Reliability as equivalence* is considered in two terms: equivalent forms and inter-rater reliability. If an equivalent form of a test or data-collecting instrument is used and yields similar results, then the instrument can be said to demonstrate this form of reliability. Here reliability can be measured through statistics (t-test), through the demonstration of a high correlation coefficient and through the demonstration of similar

means and standard deviations between two groups. If more than one researcher is taking part in a piece of research, then agreement between all researchers must be achieved (inter-rater reliability). Simply, one can calculate the inter-rater agreement as a percentage of the number of actual agreements among the number of possible agreements.

- For testing *reliability as internal consistency*, the split-half method is used. The test items are divided into two halves, ensuring that each half is matched in terms of item difficulty and content. This can be calculated using the Spearman-Brown formula: Reliability = $2r/(1+r)$, where r is the actual correlation between the halves of the instrument. An alternative measure of reliability as internal consistency is the Cronbach alpha which provides a coefficient of inter-item correlations, that is, the correlation of each item with the sum of all the other relevant items, and is useful for multi-item scales.

RELIABILITY IN QUALITATIVE RESEARCH

The premise of naturalistic qualitative studies includes the uniqueness and idiosyncrasy of situations, such that the study may not be replicated – that is their strength rather than their weakness. Denzin and Lincoln[4] suggest that reliability as replicability in qualitative research can be addressed in several ways:

- *Stability of observations*: Whether the researcher would have made the same observations and interpretation of these if they had been observed at a different time or place.
- *Parallel forms*: Whether the researchers would have made the same observations and interpretations of what had been seen if they had paid attention to other phenomena during the observation.
- *Inter-rater reliability*: Whether another observer with the same theoretical framework and observing the same phenomena would have interpreted them in the same way.

VALIDITY AND RELIABILITY OF MEASURES OF COMPETENCIES IN EDUCATIONAL RESEARCH

Competency-based assessment aims to improve the training of health care professionals in delivering consistent and high-quality patient care. This targets the 'does' level of Miller's pyramid which requires a psychometric approach such as score tests of knowledge or skill, and qualitative data such as behaviours, and attitudes across multiple domains providing more complex professional activities.[5]

Validity in the context of competency-based assessment should be the evaluation of inferences and actions that derive from a programme of assessment. Qualitative assessment data of training progression from supervisors and the learner himself from portfolios, multi-source feedback, self-assessment and reflection can be added. Five common methods are used in competency-based assessment: test, interviews, portfolios, self/peer assessment and work-based assessment.[2]

Tests[2,6]

In terms of the validity of a test, the assessment should be relevant to the competency level. Knowledge ('know how') might be measured using multiple-choice questions, modified essay questions or written examinations. 'Show how' can be measured by an objective structured clinical examination (OSCE) or mini-CEX.[6] A range of issues might affect the reliability of the test. Researchers should be concerned with factors that threaten reliability including (1) participant's factor: their motivation, concentration, health and their related skills; (2) situational factors: the psychological and physical conditions for the test; (3) test marker factors: idiosyncrasy and subjectivity and (4) instrument variables: poor domain sampling, poor question items, length of the test, mechanical errors, computer errors.

Interviews[2]

One way of validating interview measures is to compare the interview measure with another measure already shown to be valid (known as 'convergent validity'). The interviews can be more valid by minimising bias from the interviewer, the participant and the substantive content of the questions. The interviewer needs to be careful not to see the respondent in his or her own image, seek answers that support preconceived notions and to perceive what the respondent is saying. Each respondent should understand the question in the same way. The reliability of interviews can be enhanced by careful piloting of interview schedules, training of interviewers, inter-rater reliability in the coding of responses and the extended use of closed questions. The skilled interviewer promotes validity and reliability including recall and reference to earlier statements made by the participant, to clarify, confirm and modify participants' comments and allow them to take their time and answer in their own way.

Portfolios[7,8]

Portfolios are used to support reflective practice, deliver summative assessment, aid knowledge management processes and personal responsibility for learning and supporting professional development. Valuable and defensible information can be obtained during evaluation sessions, especially with respect to difficult competencies such as professionalism. Qualitative methods can be used reliably to judge portfolios. Reliability increases with more raters and with discussion between raters. Raters can agree on standards and criteria for the content and assessment of portfolios. Their reliability is enhanced by the triangulation of evidence from a number of sources. The validity of portfolios can be determined by the extent to which they document accurately those experiences that are indicators of the mastery of the desired learning outcomes.

Peer and self-assessment[5]

Peer ratings particularly have been used in the area of the assessment of attitudes and communication skills. The use of self-assessment is promising in understanding how to assess this important attribute of lifelong learning and self-discriminating abilities. Peer and self-assessment should be used in conjunction with ratings by faculty and other trained health professionals. Peer evaluations can correlate highly with faculty evaluations of the rating of the same behaviours and skills. Self-assessment correlates moderately with the rating of a trained examiner.[5] It is reported that mean ratings by self-raters tend to be lower than those of trained examiners.

Training of raters to know the provision of benchmarks, exploring standards or expected level of performance helps to improve the reliability of such ratings. The accuracy of self-assessment in clinical training may be improved by increasing the learner's awareness of the standard to be achieved. There is some indication that practical skills in clinical training may be better self-assessed than knowledge-based activities.[5]

Work-based assessment[5,8]

Work-based assessments are directly related to the practice of given tasks in daily life. Therefore, frequent formative assessment and multiple observations will be helpful in order to assess genuine skills of the practitioner and competencies required for the particular occupation. Judgements based on multiple observations by multiple assessors have strong face validity. In order to be more accurate observers and better assessors of performance, especially with respect to the complex interactions and contextual factors involved in actual patient care.[8] The agreement of assessment tools among assessors should be prepared by using clear clinical anchors, closing the gap between assessors' observation of performance and interpretation of a rating scale. For the assessors, multiple observations can be shared among the members of a properly constituted competency committee that can function legally in a 'safe place' (along the lines of peer review or morbidity meetings) to allow free discussion about the needs of individual trainees.

IN CONCLUSION

The subjective and idiosyncratic nature of the participant observation study raises questions about its external validity. How do we know that the results of this one piece of research are applicable to other situations? Fears that observers' judgements will be affected by their close involvement in the group relate to the internal validity of the method. There are several threats to validity and reliability here. For example, the researcher, in exploring the present, may be unaware of important antecedent events. The presence of the observer might bring about different behaviours (reactivity and ecological validity). The researcher might be too attached to the group disabling him to be sufficiently objective. The accuracy, objectivity, stability and repeatability of available assessment tools and methods are highly dependent on their validity and reliability. Therefore, such tools require careful review before being utilised in primary care educational research.

REFERENCES

1. Lodico MG, Spaulding DT, Voegtle KH. Measurement in educational research and assessment: preestablished instruments and archival data. In: Lodico MG, Spaulding DT, Voegtle KH, eds. *Methods in Educational Research: From Theory to Practice.* 1th ed. Jossey-Bass A Wiley Imprint: San Francisco, CA, USA 2006: 87–100.
2. Louis C, Lawrence M, Keith M. Validity and reliability. In: Louis C, Lawrence M, Keith M, eds. *Research Methods in Education.* 6th ed. New York, NY, USA: Taylor & Francis Group; 2007: 133–164.
3. Shumway JM, Harden RM. AMEE Guide No. 25: the assessment of learning outcomes for the competent and reflective physician. *Med Teach* 2003;25(6):569–584.
4. Denzin NK, Lincoln YS. *Handbook of Qualitative Research.* Sage Publications: Thousand Oaks, CA, USA. 1994.
5. Harris P, Bhanji F, Topps M, et al. Evolving concepts of assessment in a competency-based world. *Med Teach* 2017;39(6):603–608.
6. Boulet JR, Durning SJ. What we measure and what we should measure in medical education. *Med Educ* 2019;53(1):86–94.
7. Tochel C, Haig A, Hesketh A, et al. The effectiveness of portfolios for post-graduate assessment and education: BEME Guide No 12. *Med Teach* 2009;31(4):299–318.
8. Holmboe ES, Sherbino J, Long DM, Swing SR, Frank JR. The role of assessment in competency-based medical education. *Med Teach* 2010;32(8):676–682.

CHAPTER 15

Quantitative study designs

Tracie Barnett,
Jamie DeMore and
Gillian Bartlett

BACKGROUND

A great deal of research in medical education is based on the biomedical paradigm of post-positivism.[1] This ontology assumes that truth exists independently, and that there is a singular, objective reality that can be measured. Consequently, objectivity is valued, and experimental designs and methods meant to reduce subjectivity are favoured. This research paradigm employs quantitative statistical methods where we expect to generate knowledge from a sample that can be generalised to a population. The hierarchy of study designs associated with this paradigm will be recognisable to most medical education researchers from the level of evidence pyramid, where randomised control trials, the closest to pure experimental design, are seen as producing the highest levels of evidence, followed by different forms of observational study designs.[2] This chapter provides an overview of these quantitative study designs through the lens of primary care education research.

RANDOMISED CLINICAL TRIALS

In basic science, the controlled experiment is common, where all factors are held constant except for one, referred to as an independent variable or, in medical education parlance, the intervention. Typically, the experiment compares a control group against an experimental group. Everything else between the two groups is kept the same, except for the intervention being applied to be certain this 'causes' the outcome of interest. This is considered the highest possible evidence for the impact of an intervention. Obviously, when the experiment is with human participants, it is impossible and unethical to control all factors so stringently. To mimic the process of experimentation, the randomised clinical trial (RCT) method was developed.[3] In this design, the participants are 'randomised' or divided into groups by chance, and receive either the intervention being tested or a 'control'. The random allocation of participants is meant to indiscriminately distribute both known and unknown factors that might be related to the health outcome. This is expected to minimise bias caused by factors that cannot be held constant in the experiment. In this way, a well-designed trial demonstrates that the intervention 'caused' the outcome and is considered the gold standard for establishing causal conclusions.

Inclusion and exclusion criteria

Critical factors for building a high calibre RCT include inclusion and exclusion criteria, the randomisation strategy and the type of blinding that is possible.[4] Inclusion criteria usually define the characteristics of participants to be recruited for the study where the researcher would expect to see a measurable outcome, such as knowledge acquisition – normally the type of trainees[5] or participants in a specific cohort year engaging in a particular curriculum.[6] Exclusion criteria are meant to be applied to potential participants who have met all the inclusion criteria, but further restricts participation to ensure that the primary outcomes of the study are reached – this might be participants whose schedules do not fit the format of the intervention.[7] An important caveat is that the stricter the inclusion and exclusion criteria are, the less likely the researcher is able to extrapolate the evidence to a larger, more generic group of learners.

Randomisation and concealment

After participants are selected, they are randomly assigned to the intervention(s) and control group. The method of randomisation can vary from simple, such as a coin toss, to complex, with many published resources to help investigators select and complete the process.[8] A key aspect of randomisation is how allocation concealment is maintained. Allocation concealment refers to the procedures taken to ensure that the participants and the researcher are unaware to which group the participant will be randomised. This is one of the more important aspects of RCTs, so that the research team members responsible for recruitment remain impartial, in terms of which participants end up in the different intervention groups. If this does not happen, the researchers could preferentially put 'better performers' into the intervention they have developed and are trying to test.

Quasi-experimental designs are commonly used in education research when random assignment is not possible or practical, although the interpretation is not straightforward.[9,10]

Blinding

Another critical aspect is blinding or masking in the trial. Blinding refers to methods that are used to prevent study participants, researchers and/or the research team members who collect and analyse the study data from being aware of which group each participant belongs. The impact of blinding is particularly critical in education research when the outcomes are more subjective. For trials where blinding of the participants and researchers is not possible, as is often the case for interventions favoured in medical education,[11] it is still possible to blind those who are completing the data analyses. This is key for minimising bias in the measurement process.

Study design

The actual RCT design is determined by how the intervention and control groups are applied over time. Common designs are parallel, crossover, factorial and cluster.[12] While these are general descriptors of the designs, many RCTs use variations for how the intervention is applied between and across groups. Cluster randomised trials are particularly useful for education research, where interventions are more complex and difficult to apply.[11,12] For this design, complete social units or groups (clusters) are randomised to receive the intervention. This prevents contamination which might occur when an education intervention is applied within a family medicine clinic, where it is impossible to not have each other's behaviours affected. RCT designs are evolving with the complexity of interventions and many of these, such as the step-wedge cluster randomised trial, may lend themselves particularly well to education research.[11,12] An excellent and timely example of this design is in Lankin et al.'s study evaluating the impact of an internet learning module for residents.[7] While the evidence from high-quality RCTs can be compelling, it is not always ethical, feasible or possible to conduct this type of experiment. In these circumstances, observational study designs may be an option.

OBSERVATIONAL STUDIES

Observational study designs rely only on the documentation of existing information, with no manipulation on the part of the researcher. While outcomes mirror those used in experimental designs, 'exposure' is used instead of 'intervention'. *Exposure* implies a 'natural course of events' that transpire, whereas *intervention* implies a deliberate manipulation of events.

Exposures encompass both modifiable and non-modifiable individual or environmental characteristics.

Observational studies can be either descriptive or analytical. Descriptive studies provide information on patterns or levels of variables of interest, usually according to characteristics of person, place or time. In primary care education research, one could describe quality of teaching, performance or other proxies according to sex/gender, country or academic year, for example. Administrative data are sometimes re-purposed to this end. Sequist et al. used electronic medical records to describe the range and diversity of clinical experiences among medical residents in order to identify areas for curricular improvement.[13] Descriptive studies can shed light on disparities in training, performance and career opportunities, identifying opportunities to reform admissions criteria, implement curricular improvement and provide remedial strategies.

In contrast, analytic studies are conducted with specific hypotheses in mind, such as the association between types of curricula (exposure) and performance (outcome). While the collection of new data is often required, previously collected data may also be used if it is feasible, ethical and appropriate to address the research question. There are three main types of analytic study designs: cohort, case-control and cross-sectional.[14]

Cohort studies can be prospective or retrospective. In the former, participants have not yet experienced the outcome of interest. They are classified by exposure status, followed for a specified period of time, during which the outcome can be observed, or until the study ends. In a retrospective cohort study, the researcher uses existing data to define a cohort in the past. Information on variables of interest, including exposure status and any covariates, need to be available and sufficiently accurate. The cohort is then followed up administratively, i.e. also using existing data, to determine if the outcome has occurred among participants. The probability or risk of experiencing the outcome can be observed, and a relative risk can then be estimated. Often, however, information on past exposures or on important covariates is missing or insufficiently described.

Tamblyn et al. used a retrospective cohort design to investigate how exposure to a new problem-based learning curriculum impacted selected outcomes among trainees.[15] They reported indicators of performance over time in the 'exposed' students compared to 'unexposed' students (i.e. from medical schools in which the traditional curriculum was retained). A comparison group is critical, because several other factors could explain changes over time, such as admission policies. Arguably, the greatest threat to the validity of cohort studies is selection bias due to loss to follow-up. In a prospective cohort study conducted to identify risk factors for persistent burnout, surveys were sent yearly to medical residents.[16] Several possible 'exposures' or factors that might increase the risk of burnout were identified. Fewer than half of eligible respondents, however, completed questionnaires across all years, which may have compromised both the validity and generalisability of their conclusions, particularly if non-respondents differed substantially to respondents with respect to both exposure and outcome.

In a ***case-control design***, participants are selected and categorised based on whether or not they have achieved a specific outcome of interest. The crucial difference between the case-control and cohort designs is that individuals are selected and grouped on the basis of the outcome, not of the exposure. There are two common types of participant selection in case-control studies. In incidence-density case-control studies, newly occurring cases are sampled as they occur, and controls are sampled concurrently. In a cumulative incidence case-control study, cases are those that occurred over a given time period, and controls are selected at the end of the time period. Controls are selected from the same base population from which the cases arise. In one study,[17] 'cases' were defined as those who failed to complete medical school as expected, and 'controls' were graduates selected from the same academic year as the cases. Usually, the proportions of cases and controls exposed to a specific factor is compared, and a measure of association (usually the odds ratio) estimated. In some cases, comparing the intensity, length or timing of exposure may also be of interest. Case-control designs are frequently used to identify risk factors for poor performance (academic failure, lapses in professional behaviour).[17–19] Results may provide insight into the possible timing and type of intervention needed to improve outcomes, such as curricular changes or additional supervision. Case-control studies offer a time- and cost-efficient approach to answer research questions compared to cohort studies. However, because the outcome has already occurred at the time of study recruitment, outcome status may have an influence on participation and/or the information collected, leading to selection or information biases, respectively. For example, healthier cases (or controls) may be more likely to refuse (or to agree) to participate; or, cases may be more likely to 'recall' exposures than controls. If conducted correctly, using measures to minimise the potential for these biases, a case-control design can provide valid information on an association of interest.

Finally, in a ***cross-sectional study design***, both the 'exposure' status and the 'outcome' are ascertained at the same point in time. Prevalence proportions can then be compared between groups, and a prevalence ratio estimated. Interpretation may be uncertain if the sequence of occurrence of events is unclear. For example, a cross-sectional design was used to test the hypothesis that continuing medical education was associated with greater work satisfaction, but the direction of the association is unclear.[20] If temporality can be clearly established, however, then results derived from cross-sectional studies can provide valuable evidence.

Observational studies are useful to estimate associations, suggest mechanisms and inform potential strategies to address barriers.[21,22] All observational studies are susceptible to (unmeasured or poorly controlled) confounder bias, and establishing causality is challenging. Whenever possible, studies should be conceptually driven, and the availability of important covariates should be verified prior to analysis. While measurement error should be minimised in any study, it may be particularly problematic in observational studies if it is associated both with both the 'outcome' and 'exposure'; otherwise, measurement error typically biases results towards the null. Importantly, knowing who is not in the study is as important as knowing who is. A quality study will comprehensively describe the target population (i.e. to whom can we generalise our findings?), the sampling frame (i.e. from whom will we select participants?), the sample itself (i.e. who is in our study?) and, where relevant, the characteristics of those that didn't participate or were lost to follow-up. If the need for intervention is identified, any curricular, training or policy change should be tested using an experimental design before being implemented.

CONCLUSION

Quantitative study methods are appropriate to address questions when trying to answer 'what' or 'how many', using information that can be numerically measured. This process needs to be conducted as rigorously as possible, with appropriate statistical analyses and the limitations of the method acknowledged. This is a brief overview with examples of the main study designs, and each design would need to be more thoroughly investigated before embarking on any educational research.

RESOURCES
Consolidated Standards of Reporting Trials (CONSORT) http://www.consort-statement.org/Strengthening the Reporting of Observational Studies in Epidemiology (STROBE) https://www.equator-network.org/reporting-guidelines/strobe/

Online Randomisation Tools:
Study Randomizer https://app.studyrandomizer.com/
Sealed Envelope https://www.sealedenvelope.com/simple-randomiser/v1/lists
Randomizer https://www.randomizer.at/

REFERENCES

1. Phillips DC. *Postpositivism and Educational Research*. Rowman & Littlefield: Lanham, MD, USA. 2000.
2. Evans D. Hierarchy of evidence: a framework for ranking evidence evaluating healthcare interventions *J Clin Nurs* 2003;12(1):77–84.
3. Bothwell LE, Greene JA, Podolsky SH, Jones DS. Assessing the gold standard – lessons from the history of RCTs. *N Engl J Med* 2016;374(22):2175–2181.
4. Chalmers TC, Smith Jr H, Blackburn B, et al. A method for assessing the quality of a randomized control trial. *Control Clin Trials* 1981;2(1):31–49.
5. Scales Jr CD, Moin T, Fink A, et al. A randomized, controlled trial of team-based competition to increase the learner participation in quality-improvement education. *Int J Qual Health Care* 2016;28(2):227–232.
6. Cook DA, Dupras DM, Thompson WG, Pankrat VS. Web-based learning in residents' continuity clinics: a randomized, controlled trial. *Acad Med* 2005;80(1):90–97.
7. Lanken PN, Novack DH, Daetwyler C, et al. Efficacy of an internet-based learning module and small-group debriefing on trainees' attitudes and communication skills toward patients with substance use disorders: results of a cluster randomized controlled trial. *Acad Med* 2015;90(3):345–54.
8. Suresh KP. An overview of randomization techniques: an unbiased assessment of outcome in clinical research *J Hum Reprod Sci* 2001;4(1):8.
9. Janson SL, Cooke M, Wong McGrath K, Kroon LA, Robinson S, Baron RB. Improving chronic care of type 2 diabetes using teams of interprofessional learners. *Acad Med* 2009;84(11):1540–1548.
10. Gribbons B, Herman J. True and quasi-experimental designs. *Pract Assess Res Eval* 1996;5(1):1–3.
11. Thompson C, Kinmonth AL, Stevens L, et al. Effects of a clinical-practice guideline and practice-based education on detection and outcome of depression in primary care: Hampshire Depression Project randomised controlled trial *Lancet* 2000;335:185–191.
12. Bartlett G, Dickinson M, Schuster T. Randomised controlled trials in primary care. In: Goodyear-Smith F, Mash B, eds. *How To Do Primary Care Research*. CRC Press-Taylor & Francis; 2018: 203–212.
13. Sequist TD, Singh S, Pereira AG, Rusinak D, Pearson SD. Use of an electronic medical record to profile the continuity clinic experiences of primary care residents. *Acad Med* 2005;80(4):390–394.
14. Kelsey JL. *Methods in Observational Epidemiology*. New York: Oxford University Press; 1996.
15. Tamblyn R, Abrahamowicz M, Dauphinee D, et al. Effect of a community oriented problem based learning curriculum on quality of primary care delivered by graduates: historical cohort comparison study. *BMJ* 2005;331(7523):1002.
16. Campbell J, Prochazka AV, Yamashita T, Gopal R. Predictor of persistent burnout in internal medicine residents: a prospective cohort study. *Acad Med* 2010;85(10):1630–1634.
17. Yates J, James D. Predicting the "strugglers": a case-control study of students at Nottingham University Medical School. *BMJ* 2006;332:1009.
18. Klamen DL, Borgia PT. Can students' scores on preclerkship clinical perfromance examinations predict that they will fail a senior clinical performance examination? *Acad Med* 2011;86(4):516–520.
19. Hoffman LA, Shew RL, Vu R, Brokaw JJ, Frankel RM. Is reflective ability associated with professionalism lapses in medical school? *Acad Med* 2016;91(6):853–857.
20. Kushnir T, Cohen AH, Kitai E. Continuing medical education and primary physicians' job stress, burnout and dissatisfaction. *Med Educ* 2000;34:430–436.

21. Jagsi R, Griffith KA, Jones RD, Stewart A, Ubel PA. Factors associated with success of clinician-researchers receiving career development awards from the national institutes of health: a longitudinal cohort study. *Acad Med* 2017;92(10):1429–1439.
22. Reed DA, Enders F, Lindor R, McClees M, Lindor KD. Gender differences in academic productivity and leadership appointments of physicians throughout academic careers. *Acad Med* 2011;86(1):43–47.

CHAPTER 16

Big data in primary care educational research

Jon Dowell

THE POTENTIAL OF BIG DATA

Big data, by which we mean primarily routine data, collated systematically and over time, on more than one school, college or institution can change the way we approach research in medical education. This is an area that is destined to grow as data becomes more available and is important for primary care, in particular to inform workforce planning. This chapter addresses why we need big data, the types of studies it enables and what may be unlocked in the longer term.

WHY DO WE NEED BIG DATA?

Medical education is extremely expensive, in both financial and human terms, so it should have proportional research and development activity employing all sources of information available. However, our sources of rich routine data, such as those used in selection, assessment and progression systems, are rarely systematically linked. Conducting research over time, involving more than a few sources or time points is costly, but enhances our capacity in many ways to understand the impact of change, such as new medical schools or educational approaches.

This is a complex area, as data protection and sharing issues abound alongside 'ownership' issues and institutional concerns about reputational impact. The challenge of establishing buy-in, collating and using data should not be underestimated. However, where achieved these have proved very productive, examples include Jefferson Medical School,[1] New York University,[2] Medical

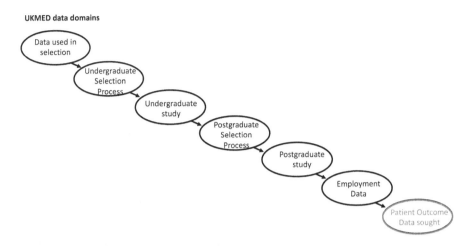

UKMED data domains

FIGURE 16.1 Individual-level data held in UKMED.

Schools Outcomes Database[3] and more recently the United Kingdom Medical Education Database (UKMED).[4] This latter data source is used as an example.

UK MEDICAL EDUCATION DATABASE

Key features

The UKMED was launched in 2015 as a joint General Medical Council (GMC) and the Medical Schools Council Initiative. This combination of the regulator's authority, drivers and resources, along with broad academic involvement, has overcome the challenges and built an openly accessible data repository with associated safeguards. UKMED has collated information on all UK medical school entrants from 2003 onwards, including most of the key important data points. Figure 16.1 depicts the individual-level data held for students/graduates which, in 2020, included 210,000 applications to medical school, 135,000 student and 49,000 postgraduate subjects, with metrics such as socioeconomic and secondary school grades, graduation and postgraduate exam information in all specialities, job application data and career history.[4]

Uses

The potential from this growing repository for data extraction is immense, with nine studies published to date, and over 30 others underway (UKMED[5]). Examples:

1. *Recruitment to specialties with shortages, including primary care.* Doctors with certain demographic backgrounds and educational factors have been found more likely to apply for general practice (GP) training, supporting

the case for widening student participation.[6] This has helped inform the allocation of extra medical student places.

2. *Rare events*. Concerns about 'Fitness to Practice' are rare but important. UKMED has revealed that white ethnicity and UK nationality are associated with increased odds of both conduct and health-related declarations, whilst students from non-professional backgrounds are at increased risk of depression.[7]

3. *Selection*. The impact of independent or state schooling has been quantified, contributing to the debate about justifiable contextual adjustment in medical school selection.[8]

4. *External data*. Identifiable data from other sources can be added to enable long-term follow-up, such as the Conscientiousness Index predictive validity postgraduation.[9]

5. *Equity* is important yet complex. Gender variation between medical specialties has been shown to be primarily due to differential application, although men are also less likely to be offered or accept a place in GP.[10]

Challenges

A word of caution. The UKMED was four years in planning, is largely resourced by the GMC and has extensive safeguards requiring researchers to work within a safe haven to ensure data protection. It is complex to run, partly to ensure data cannot be used for decisions about individuals and a clear governance framework oversees studies. Institutional tracking systems (e.g. Jefferson and New York Universities) are simpler, and can utilise finer grained data. For instance, a local change in selection approaches or clinical attachments might be tracked via graduate questionnaires. They may also be constructed to link with other to additional tracking studies if considered at the design phase (e.g. gaining consent and retaining identifiers). If planning to create a data repository, starting locally will be more achievable, but looking ahead with potential future collaborators or national bodies is advisable.

TYPES OF STUDIES

This section explores the pros and cons of alternative approaches.

Local data

Systematically collating local data over time (selection, performance, sociodemographic and other data) in a manner that are retrievable and accessible is far simpler and still has great potential, especially if linkable with additional sources such as bespoke surveys. The impact of selection approaches on primary care career preference might be tracked, as changes to the style or quantity of primary care educational experience can affect this, but this would require a follow-up system or surveys.

Collaborative

Organisations that collaborate and align their data have opportunity to do comparative studies, increase the value to others and thereby enhance research opportunities. For example, UKCAT12, a collaborative work with 12 medical schools.[11]

Comprehensive

Data collation across many institutions, over time and bridging undergraduate-postgraduate studies, offer the most promise. The complexities can be overcome, the information will be coarser grained, as only common metrics are manageable and comparable. Even then, there is a need to track and manage 'metadata' carefully, so that changes over time are captured. For instance, the impact of COVID-19 on selection and assessments globally means this cohort's data are atypical.

Despite the challenges, if we are ever to truly know if more women, graduate entrants or empathic interviewees are going to cultivate more, or more resilient or better family doctors, then we should seek to develop multiple big data resources internationally.

THE FUTURE

Looking ahead, what might these types of datasets lead to or support? Some of the most exciting suggestions include:

- *Collaborative research programmes* designed to optimise specific aspects of practice, such as refining selection tools and their impact on the graduates produced.
- *Comparative studies* that can probe the difference between the graduates produced by traditional, systems-based, case-based or problem-based programmes through comparing adequate numbers from contrasting schools.
- *Trials* where institutions collaborate on introducing common changes, particularly where the outcome is rare. Can selection or resilience 'training' reduce future Fitness to Practice concerns or the incidence of burnout in graduates?
- Ongoing affordable long-term *workforce and career pathway studies*.

The ideal, which is becoming achievable, is to link with patient care outcomes using the emerging clinician-level data in areas such as surgical outcomes, prescribing, patient satisfaction, etc. to assess if training, exam grades or other factors can make a difference.[12]

Returning to the enormous investment medical education represents, surely it is time to capitalise on big data systematically, to combine forces and bring its power to the cause. Such important questions justify the effort and for the sake of educators' scholarly base, doctors' learning and even patient care. It is time to push for this. There is now clear evidence doing so is productive, and big data collections will therefore also support educators' careers, an indirect but important benefit.

REFERENCES

1. Jefferson Medical School. Available from: https://www.jefferson.edu/academics/colleges-schools-institutes/skmc/research/research-medical-education/longitudinal-study-medical-education.html (Accessed 14 August 2021).
2. New York University. Available from: https://med.nyu.edu/prmeir/collaborations/database-research-education-academic-medicine (Accessed 14 August 2021).
3. Medical Schools Outcomes Database. Available from: https://medicaldeans.org.au/data/medical-schools-outcomes-database-reports/ (Accessed 14 August 2021).
4. Dowell J, Cleland J, Fitzpatrick S, et al. The UK medical education database (UKMED) what is it? Why and how might you use it? *BMC Med Educ* 2018;18:6. doi:10.1186/s12909-017-1115-9
5. United Kingdom Medical Education Database. Available from: https://www.ukmed.ac.uk (Accessed 14/9/2021)
6. Gale T, Lambe P, Roberts M. Factors associated with junior doctors' decisions to apply for general practice training programmes in the UK: secondary analysis of data from the UKMED project. *BMC Med* 2017;15(1):220. doi:10.1186/s12916-017-0982-6.
7. Paton L, Tiffin P, Smith D, Dowell J, Mwandigha L. Predictors of fitness to practise declarations in UK medical undergraduates. *BMC Med Educ* 2018;18(1):68. doi:10.1186/s12909-018-1167-5.
8. Kumwenda B, Cleland J, Walker K, Lee A, Greatrix R. The relationship between school type and academic performance at medical school: a national, multi-cohort study. *BMJ Open* 2017;7(8): e016291. doi:10.1136/bmjopen-2017-016291.
9. Kelly M, O'Flynn S, McLachlan J, Sawdon M. The clinical conscientiousness index. *Acad Med* 2012;87(9):1218–1224. doi:10.1097/ACM.0b013e3182628499
10. Woolf K, Jayaweera H, Unwin E, et al. Effect of sex on specialty training application outcomes: a longitudinal administrative data study of UK medical graduates. *BMJ Open* 2019;9:e025004. doi:10.1136/bmjopen-2018-025004
11. McManus C, Dewry C, Nicholson S, Dowell J. The UKCAT-12 study: educational attainment, aptitude test performance, demographic and socio-economic contextual factors as predictors of first year outcome in a collaborative study of twelve UK medical schools. *BMC Med* 2013;11:244. doi:10.1186/1741-7015-11-244. Available from: http://www.biomedcentral.com/1741-7015/11/244
12. Tamblyn R, Abrahamowicz M, Brailovsky C, et al. Association between licensing examination scores and resource use and quality of care in primary care practice. *JAMA* 1998;280(11):989–996. doi:10.1001/jama.280.11.989

CHAPTER 17

Social media and the internet in primary care educational research

Charilaos Lygidakis, Vincent Kalumire Cubaka and Raquel Gómez Bravo

Internet-based tools and social networking sites are frequently used by both students and health care professionals with the purpose of engaging with communities, collecting and sharing information and learning.[1]

For example, technology has enabled the surge of virtual communities of practice. Communities of practice are established when there is a common learning interest on a subject, and intention to share experience and knowledge through regular interactions and collaborative activities with the use of a mutually agreed set of resources and tools.[2,3] Researchers can help establish such communities, or approach already-existing ones to recruit participants and carry out different types of studies (e.g. qualitative or quantitative, observational or experimental). Learning management systems (such as the open-source Moodle and Open edX), in addition to offering tools to host, manage and localise content, can also help with the creation of communities of learners. With such platforms, teachers can arrange assessments and manage participants, including running courses and evaluations for specific cohorts.

Social networking sites and mobile devices have enabled the creation of informal communities to address unmet needs (e.g. groups on Facebook, Slack, WhatsApp, Telegram). Furthermore, communities of practice can benefit from a blended approach, combining real-time (in-place or virtual) activities with asynchronous, distant and most often computer-facilitated learning (for instance, pre-recorded lectures, slideshows, podcasts).[4,5] Such techniques also allow interprofessional training which can be particularly beneficial in the case of primary care.

PLANNING AHEAD AND LIMITATIONS

When conducting educational research, it is necessary to plan the recruitment and engagement strategy, as institutional review boards and ethics committees typically require evaluation of methods and techniques, including proposed advertisement messages and compliance with the network's terms of use. Advertising on general social networking sites is a cost-effective recruitment strategy which can be continuously monitored and fine-tuned; however, the appropriate network(s) should be selected depending on the research objectives and targeted population. Researchers must be transparent and concise in their online communication and, before employing such tools, be aware of some caveats, such as the possibilities of self-selection and sampling bias limiting generalisability of the results, mismatch between target population and type of social media network and contamination due to communication among participants.

In addition to well-known limitations, such as connectivity and compatibility of software and information systems, there are other barriers which can undermine the use of mobile devices to support educational research: distraction due to social connectivity or other personal uses, disapproval from supervisors or peers, concerns related to confidentiality and privacy, security issues and unclear or inconsistent messages regarding policy.[6-8] Hindrances in the integration of social media at the institutional level for educational and research purposes resemble those identified when adopting blended learning strategies (e.g. unwritten rules and expectations, accreditation, hierarchy).[9,10]

SOFTWARE FOR CONDUCTING RESEARCH

For observational studies, public social media data (e.g. available from educational communities on Twitter) can be retrieved and interpreted with relatively affordable tools such as NodeXL which can help with the calculation of metrics and content analysis, clustering messages and mapping their relationships.

A plethora of internet-based software is available to researchers to cover their various needs at prices they can afford. Notably, such software can help improve collaboration in multicentric projects. Although many solutions require a dedicated server, in recent years, more developers are offering cloud-based Software-as-a-Service (SaaS) with different subscription types. Investigators who focus on educational research can use survey software, such as Limesurvey and SoSci Survey.

RESEARCH DISSEMINATION

Digital technologies are providing opportunities for innovative research dissemination and knowledge translation. Beyond the traditional research dissemination vehicles like printed academic journals, books, conferences and workshops, researchers are embracing a variety of new digital tools including online journals, e-books, social media, blogs and wikis.[11] These tools have made research accessible to a wider audience, including researchers, patients, clinicians, policy-makers and general public.[12] Furthermore, they have proven to facilitate research understanding, uptake, feedback, engagement, collaboration and have ultimately increased social impact. They are open, interactive and encourage participation, therefore aligned with modern educational theories.[13] A topical example can be seen in how social media and other digital technologies are helping fight the COVID-19 pandemic through rapid and effective dissemination of knowledge, raising awareness and influencing policies, practices and behaviours.[14]

The following rules can be recommended for embracing and leveraging responsible use of digital tools with the aim of communicating primary care educational research. These rules are adapted from the "ten steps to innovative dissemination".[11,15]

1. Start with the basics of dissemination:
   - Define the objectives: what do you want to achieve with your dissemination?
   - Map the audience: who do you want your research results to reach and for which purposes?
   - Target and frame the key message: consider the audience's perspective. What could they want or need to hear from me?
   - Define the communication channel: the communication medium will depend on the objectives.
   - Formulate a dissemination plan: this is often a requirement for research proposals. The plan will help set milestones, assign roles, define activities and allocate a budget. The plan should be adaptable to changes in research directions.

2. Develop a strong online profile to make you and your research visible. Use personal websites, social media (e.g. Facebook, Twitter, LinkedIn, Instagram, SlideShare, YouTube), researcher identifiers (e.g. ORCID) and academic social networks (e.g. ResearchGate, Academia.edu, Google Scholar).

3. Engage with the audience, for example, by sharing frequent updates on a blog or Twitter.

4. Foster open science for greater impact through more transparency, replicability, participation, collaboration and knowledge access and reuse.[16]
5. Disseminate traditional research outputs through digital media: to better reach your target audiences and boost impact.
6. Consider innovative live events like science festivals, science slams, Science Shops and TEDx talks.
7. Use quality visuals to help your audience better understand, retain and interpret your research.[17]
8. Respect diversity by being inclusive in the dissemination to reach all those concerned.
9. Find innovative dissemination resources. Use catalogues of dissemination tools and services.
10. Assess your dissemination activities and their impact: Are they having the expected impact? If not, why not?

REFERENCES

1. Arnbjörnsson E. The use of social media in medical education: a literature review. *Creat Educ* 2014;5(24):2057–2061. doi:10.4236/ce.2014.524229
2. Wenger E. *Communities of Practice: Learning, Meaning, and Identity. Syst Thinker.* Cambridge, UK: Cambridge University Press; 1999: 318p.
3. Lave J, Wenger E. *Situated Learning : Legitimate Peripheral Participation. Learning in doing.* Cambridge England; New York: Cambridge University Press; 1991: 138p.
4. Barnett S, Jones SC, Caton T, Iverson D, Bennett S, Robinson L. Implementing a virtual community of practice for family physician training: a mixed-methods case study. *J Med Internet Res* 2014;16(3):e83. Available from: http://www.ncbi.nlm.nih.gov/pubmed/24622292
5. Lygidakis H, McLoughlin C, Patel K. *Achieving Universal Health Coverage: Technology for innovative primary health care education.* World Organization of Family Doctors (WONCA), 2016. Available from: https://issuu.com/iheed/docs/ict4uhcreport
6. Ellaway R. The informal and hidden curricula of mobile device use in medical education. *Med Teach* 2014;36(1):89–91. doi:10.3109/0142159X.2014.862426
7. Ellaway RH, Fink P, Graves L, Campbell A. Left to their own devices: medical learners' use of mobile technologies. *Med Teach* 2014;36(2):130–138. doi:10.3109/0142159X.2013.849800
8. Hafferty FW. Beyond curriculum reform: confronting medicine's hidden curriculum. *Acad Med.* 1998 Apr;73(4):403–407.
9. Shelton C. Giving up technology and social media: why university lecturers stop using technology in teaching. *Technol Pedagog Educ* 2017;26(3):303–321. doi:10.1080/1475939X.2016.1217269
10. Keenan ID, Slater JD, Matthan J. Social media: insights for medical education from instructor perceptions and usage. *MedEdPublish* 2018;7(1):27. doi:10.15694/mep.2018.0000027.1
11. Ross-Hellauer T, Tennant JP, Banelytė V, et al. Ten simple rules for innovative dissemination of research. *PLOS Comput Biol* 2020;16(4):1–12. doi:10.1371/journal.pcbi.1007704

12. Allen HG, Stanton TR, Di Pietro F, Moseley GL. Social media release increases dissemination of original articles in the clinical pain sciences. *PLOS ONE* 2013;8(7):1–6. doi:10.1371/journal.pone.0068914

13. Cooper A. The use of online strategies and social media for research dissemination in education. *Educ Policy Anal Arch* 2014;22:88. doi:10.14507/epaa.v22n88.2014.

14. Chan AKM, Nickson CP, Rudolph JW, Lee A, Joynt GM. Social media for rapid knowledge dissemination: early experience from the COVID-19 pandemic. *Anaesthesia* 2020. 75(12):1579–1582. doi:10.1111/anae.15057

15. Bik HM, Dove ADM, Goldstein MC, et al. Ten simple rules for effective online outreach. *PLOS Comput Biol* 2015;11(4):1–8. doi:10.1371/journal.pcbi.1003906

16. Vicente-Saez R, Martinez-Fuentes C. Open Science now: a systematic literature review for an integrated definition. *J Bus Res* 2018;88:428–436. Available from: http://www.sciencedirect.com/science/article/pii/S0148296317305441

17. Martin LJ, Turnquist A, Groot B, et al. Exploring the role of infographics for summarizing medical literature. *Heal Prof Educ* 2019;5(1):48–57. doi:10.1016/j.hpe.2018.03.005

CHAPTER 18

Use of the Delphi technique in educational research

Felicity Goodyear-Smith

HISTORY OF THE DELPHI TECHNIQUE

The Delphi process derives its name from Greek mythology. Delphi was the site of the major oracle of Apollo, from where he made most of his prophecies. The Delphi technique was developed by the RAND Corporation in the 1960s as a forecasting methodology.[1] It is a tool based on the three characteristics of anonymity, statistical analysis and feedback of reasoning which allows a group of experts to reach a consensus of opinion. The technique involves asking a panel of experts to take part anonymously in a series of rounds to clarify, refine and gain consensus on a particular issue. As the panel do not meet, individuals can express their opinion without being influenced by others, and only the moderator (researcher) is aware of their identity. The process is structured and iterative.

WHEN TO USE THE DELPHI TECHNIQUE?

This method is valuable when expert opinions are sought on a question for which there is no absolute answer, and a collective subjective judgement is required.[2] It enables engaging a number of people, sometimes from varied backgrounds, experience and expertise, where number or location of participants, time and cost make face-to-face interactions infeasible. It allows for arbitration of disagreements, to ensure a consistent message is disseminated when a united public front is required. A valid collective result hence is generated without domination from a strong personality or group ('bandwagon effect').

The technique is particularly useful in areas of uncertainty and complexity, where possible future scenarios are explored collectively, leading to a planned coordinated action. Through participating in several rounds, panellists can gain knowledge about a problem and reflect on the issues before developing a concerted approach.

SELECTION OF YOUR PANEL

The panel of experts you choose directly influences the quality of your results. You need to select them carefully. The Delphi method aims to provide an in-depth insight into a complex issue, but is not intended for generalisation of results.[3] An 'expert' should have first-hand experience and knowledge of the area in question, be able to make a useful contribution and be prepared to give the time to adequately participate. Other criteria might include participants self-rating themselves as experts in the topic, or based on a review of their scientific publications. There is no fixed number for a panel, and this depends on the context and aim of your study. It has been suggested that if your experts have extended knowledge of the topic, 10–15 may be sufficient.[3]

NUMBER OF ROUNDS

In general, there are two to six rounds, and three structured rounds are generally sufficient.[4] Participants might cease to engage and drop out when there are multiple rounds,[3] and some researchers have found there is little improvement on insights after three rounds.[2] In a modified technique, you can also use a 'pre-Delphi' round, using open-ended questions to generate the material around which you then seek consensus. For example, this might be generating a list of research questions that the panel then prioritises,[5] determining key learning outcomes for students (see Box 18.1)[6] or deciding on the core outcomes to be used in a proposed trial.[7]

ANALYSES

Free-text pre-Delphi data can undergo qualitative analysis to determine the factors around which you then seek to gain consensus from the panel. Decide what constitutes consensus – often considered to be 80% agreement. The median with the inter-quartile range and response spread can be used to determine consensus, or alternatively the collective priorities can be determined through the order in which they are ranked.

GUIDANCE ON CONDUCTING AND REPORTING ON DELPHI STUDIES

Like all research methods, this technique had both advantages and limitations (see Table 18.1). Specific Guidance on Conducting and REporting DElphi Studies (CREDES) can be found at https://www.equator-network.org/reporting-guidelines/credes/. This covers a number of items including justifying your choice of this method, panel section, defining consensus, prevention of bias and interpretation and reporting of results.

BOX 18.1 EXAMPLE OF USE IN PRIMARY CARE EDUCATION RESEARCH

Our aim was to develop common rural-specific learning outcomes for four different medical student regional-rural programmes.[6] Our panel consisted of all the rural hospital doctors and general practitioners who were clinical teachers on these programmes. In a pre-Delphi round, participants were asked to generate up to 10 explicit rural learning outcomes, with a list of verbs based on Bloom's taxonomy to guide them. Their suggestions were collated, analysed by themes using a general inductive approach, sorted by codes, collapsed and synthesised into a list of key learning outcomes. In the first true Delphi round, panellists rated each outcome for importance on a Likert scale. Collated responses were ordered in degree of importance. In the final round, the learning outcomes were ranked by 'drag and drop' into order of importance, and the top four were selected as the primary learning outcomes for the programmes.

TABLE 18.1 Advantages and pitfalls[8]

Advantages	Pitfalls and Limitations
Builds consensus	There may be group pressure to reach consensus
Can bring experts from different locations and time zones together	No established guidelines for sample size
Participants given limited time to complete each survey	Participants need to commit time for each round
Responses are anonymous and confidential	Results are opinion-based not analytical
Avoids direct conflict between participants and encourages honest opinion	May force 'middle-of-the road' consensus
Structured group communication process	Selection issues: not all panellists may be true 'experts' on the topic
Valid as content driven by panellists	Results may have limited reliability
Reduces the 'bandwagon' effect	Anonymity may be a disadvantage when the source of a statement is more significant than its substance
Cost-effective and flexible	
Simple to use	
Valuable to provide new data where there is uncertainty or imperfect knowledge	

CONCLUSION

The Delphi technique is another tool that can be useful in primary care educational research. It can help in forming guidelines, setting standards and predicting trends.[9] It works well as an initial planning step, and can be used in curriculum development, and establishing educational goals and objectives. It can also be used with students for their assessment and feedback on the curriculum, where they may be hesitant to speak out in interviews or focus groups. This technique lends itself to use in situations where there is no one answer, but critical examination and discussion are required, and decision-making based on informed sound judgement.

REFERENCES

1. Dalkey N, Helmer-Hirschberg O. An experimental application of the Delphi method to the use of experts. *Manage Sci* 1963;9(3):351–515.
2. Linstone H, Turnoff M. *The Delphi Method: Techniques and Applications*. Newark, NJ, USA: Addison-Wesley Publishing Company; 2002.
3. Alarabiat A, Ramos I. The Delphi method research in information systems research (2004-2017). *EJBRM* 2019;17(2):86–99. doi:34190/JBRM.17.2.04
4. Skinner R, Nelson R, Chin W, et al. The Delphi method research strategy in studies of information system. *Commun Assoc Inf Syst* 2015;37(2):31–63. doi:10.17705/1CAIS.03702
5. Goodyear-Smith F, Bazemore A, Coffman M, et al. Primary care research priorities in low-and middle-income countries. *Ann Fam Med* 2019;17(1):31–35. doi:10.1370/afm.2329
6. Eggleton K, Wearn A, Goodyear-Smith F. Determining rural learning outcomes for medical student placements using a consensus process with rural clinical teachers. *Educ Prim Care* 2020;31(1):24–31. doi:10.1080/14739879.2019.1705921
7. Sinha IP, Smyth RL, Williamson PR. Using the Delphi technique to determine which outcomes to measure in clinical trials: recommendations for the future based on a systematic review of existing studies. *PLoS Med* 2011;8(1):e1000393–e93. doi:10.1371/journal.pmed.1000393
8. Hung HL, Altschuld JW, Lee YF. Methodological and conceptual issues confronting a cross-country Delphi study of educational program evaluation. *Eval Program Plann* 2008;31(2):191–198. doi:10.1016/j.evalprogplan.2008.02.005
9. Green RA. The Delphi technique in educational research. *SAGE Open* 2014;4(2):1–8. doi:10.1177/2158244014529773

CHAPTER 19

Qualitative methods

Charo Rodriguez

The term qualitative research encompasses those systematic inquiry processes through which investigators aim to generate new knowledge about what and why people think and behave, and how they give meaning to what they live in their naturally occurring settings.[1] Emerging from social sciences, qualitative research is a complex field of inquiry that sits across research paradigms, disciplines, fields and subject matter.[1]

Qualitative research has progressively been adopted and legitimated in medical and health professions education, including primary care education research. Qualitative researchers count on an array of methods for gathering (or generating) and analysing data. Qualitative data is basically constituted by texts, broadly understood as communicative events in which linguistic, cognitive and social actions converge, and through which the world is understood.[2] Methods are those tools that will enable the development of an empirical study. Congruent with the nature of qualitative research, qualitative methods must be flexible and sensitive to the social and cultural contexts in which they are applied. Importantly, methods do not stand by themselves, but are used in coherence with researchers' beliefs and preferences at the ontological, epistemological and methodological levels, and the research question they want to answer.

This chapter offers an overview of a number of these tools, and the way they might be used in a qualitative research project that aspires to advance knowledge in the field of primary care education.

REALITY, KNOWLEDGE AND PROCEDURES OF INQUIRY

To ensure a strong research design, researchers must choose a research paradigm that is congruent with their beliefs about the nature of reality. Consciously subjecting such beliefs to an ontological interrogation in the first instance will illuminate the epistemological and methodological possibilities that are available.[3]

First coined by Thomas Kuhn is his seminal work, *The Structure of Scientific Revolutions*,[4] a research paradigm is a rather elusive term[5] that refers to the consensual set of beliefs, principles and actions akin to a community of research practice. Ontology, epistemology and methodology are the three major intertwined components of research paradigms, and together provide coherent philosophical foundations for the different worldviews or basic belief systems 'that guide disciplined inquiry'.[6] There are many, the literature having reported tensions among the tenants of one or another.[7] As it is the case in other areas of knowledge, what currently characterises the field of education research is the use of a variety of paradigms that range from more traditional positivist and postpositivist through interpretive and constructivist to pragmatic, critical and participatory perspectives.[8] This plurality is also present regarding methodological approaches.[8] In qualitative studies, the available set of methods for collecting and analysing qualitative data will be used differently, in congruency to the research paradigm that frames the investigation, the research question to be answered and the methodological perspective adopted.

METHODS FOR GENERATING QUALITATIVE DATA
Interviews

Qualitative interviewing is the most recognised and used method for generating qualitative data.[9] Echoing 'a long tradition in social science', Burgess views qualitative interviews as 'conversations with a purpose'.[10] This technique is used when people's thoughts, behaviours, experiences and interpretations are meaningful features of the reality about which the researcher wants to generate new knowledge.[11] At the epistemological level, the researcher also assumes that talking is an appropriate means for producing data about the issue at stake. Qualitative interviews can range from in-depth through semi-structured to more loosely structured forms of interviewing. They can also adopt different styles, e.g. narrative, biographical, ethnographic, thematic. Traditionally conducted in person, qualitative interviews can also be held by phone,[12] and online interviews are of increasing interest nowadays.[13]

An important distinction exists between individual and group interviews in which the researcher meets with more than one participant. In individual interviews, data emerge from the more or less structured and in-depth interaction between the participant and the researcher. In group interviews which can also adopt a variety of modalities (from very structured expert consensus panels such as Nominal and Delphi groups, through deliberative public methods, rather semi-structured focus groups, to natural groups), data are basically produced in the interaction among participants, the researcher adopting a role of moderator or facilitator.[14]

The different modalities of qualitative interviewing share the need for the researcher to scrupulously plan and conduct the encounters. This includes the acquisition of necessary knowledge and skills for the researcher to become a qualified qualitative interviewer, the preparation of the interview guideline, selection of participants, organisation of the events and awareness of ethical issues related to the interview interaction.[9,11]

Observations

According to the Oxford Dictionary, to observe is to 'notice or perceive (something) and register it as being significant'. Having its grounds in anthropology, and usually associated with ethnography, observations constitute a privilege tool for the qualitative researcher who aims to get insight about people's behaviours, interactions, events and any other phenomenon relative to the topic being examined in their naturally occurring contexts.[15] Observations can range from unstructured to structured, but it is always convenient for the researcher to create a checklist to help remember what to observe during fieldwork.

Consistent with the research paradigm, methodology and research question to be answered, and being aware of all the ethical challenges, it is essential that researchers are aware and reflect on the different possible observer roles to adopt during fieldwork: from complete participant, through participant-as-observer and observer-as-participant, to complete observer.[16] It is important to identify key informants – individuals who can be good sources of information about the issue being examined. Qualitative researchers record the observations performed, and their own experiences during fieldwork, commonly known as field notes, written during or immediately after the observations.

Documents

Documents constitute another valuable source of empirical material in qualitative research. Green and Thorogood define documents at those 'whole range of written and material sources that might be available relating to a topic, but which were not created by the researcher specifically for their study'.[17] Lincoln and Guba distinguish between 'document' and 'record'[18]: a record is any piece of written or recorded material created with the aim to attesting to something, e.g. birth, marriage and death records; minutes of meetings. Documents are all written or recorded materials that are not records, e.g. letters, diaries, newspaper editorials. Generally used in combination with other methods for generating qualitative data, and particularly pertinent to gather information about context, document analysis involves a systematic process through which the researcher must not only find and select, but also appraise and synthesise data in documents in relation to the issue being studied.[19]

METHODS FOR ANALYSING QUALITATIVE DATA

Qualitative data analysis has been defined as 'the classification and interpretation of linguistic (or visual) material to make statements about implicit and explicit dimensions and structures of meaning-making in the material and what is represent in it'.[20] The paradigmatic position in which researchers are framed matters in relation to the ways they perform qualitative data analysis. For a postpositivist qualitative researcher, qualitative data analysis implies the answer to the question: 'How can we draw valid meaning from qualitative data?'[21] For a more interpretive/constructivist researcher, this question would be stated 'How to construct and present a convincing explanation or argument on the basis of qualitative data?'[9]

Qualitative data analysis is always a key piece of the puzzle, and a recursive rather than longitudinal procedure. Either from a deductive, inductive or hybrid perspective, qualitative data analysis needs to be planned carefully at the outset of the investigation in terms of type and volume of data to be generated, how it will be stored and eventually shared, the specific techniques to be used for data analysis, identifying the researchers who will perform data analysis and what will be done with data once the study is finished.[9]

Several techniques can help the researcher to make sense to the empirical material generated in a qualitative study. Two of these are content analysis and thematic analysis. Content analysis labels a set of techniques used to systematically examine verbal, visual or written data to describe the phenomenon at stake. Quantitative content analysis allows for the quantification of the occurrence of words, phrases or any unit of analysis determined by the researcher, whereas qualitative content analysis can focus on the description of the subject matter of the text.[22]

A widely used tool for analysing qualitative data is thematic analysis. This method entails the identification, interpretation and report of patterns (recurrent ideas), called themes, within the corpus of data.[23] Adopting different modalities such as deductive, inductive, semantic, latent, thematic analysis involves a series of interrelated phases. For Braun and Clarke,[23] thematic analysis first requires the researcher to familiarise with the data, then search for themes and generate initial codes, followed by the review of themes, finishing with the definition and naming of resulting themes and production of the findings report.

CONCLUSION

This chapter briefly outlines those most common methods for collecting and analysing qualitative data. Other chapters in this book further develop some of the pieces here just sketched. Chapter 2 discusses the ontological, epistemological and methodological underpinnings of primary care education research. Case studies, action research and ethnography, three major methodological approaches in education, are covered in Chapters 20, 21 and 24, respectively. A narrative opposing individual interviews and focus groups is offered in Chapter 22. The Delphi technique is presented in Chapter 18, and content analysis introduced in Chapter 23.

Qualitative research is a very rich field of inquiry that offers multitude of opportunities for researchers to meaningfully conduct primary care education research. Qualitative methods for collecting and analysing qualitative empirical material are key elements of this research enterprise. More specifically, they are those tools or techniques that allow the researcher to conduct qualitative empirical investigations. When aspiring to conduct sound qualitative research, methods never stand by themselves: their selection and use should always be congruent with the researcher's paradigmatic position, the phenomenon being examined, the methodology adopted and the research question to be answered.

REFERENCES

1. Denzin NK, Lincoln YS. Introduction: the discipline and practice of qualitative research. In: Denzin NK, Lincoln YS, eds. *Strategies of Qualitative Inquiry.* 3rd ed. Thousand Oaks, CA: Sage; 2008: 1–43.
2. Jurin S, Krišković A. *Texts and Their Usage Through Text Linguistic and Cognitive Linguistic Analysis.* Rijeka: Faculty of Humanities and Social Sciences; 2017.
3. Mills J, Bonner A, Francis K. The development of constructivist grounded theory. *Int J Qual Methods* 2006;5(1):25–35.
4. Kuhn T. *The Structure of Scientific Revolutions.* Chicago, IL: University of Chicago Press; 1962.
5. Donmoyer R. Take my paradigm...please! The legacy of Kuhn's construct in educational research. *Int J Qual Stud Educ* 2006;19(1):1–10.
6. Guba EG. *The Paradigm Dialog.* Newbury Park: Sage; 1990.
7. Lincoln YS, Guba EG. Paradigmatic controversies, contradictions, and emerging confluences. In: Denzin NK, Lincoln YS, eds. *The SAGE Handbook of Qualitative Research.* 5th ed. Thousand Oaks, CA: Sage; 2017: 163–188.
8. Cohen L, Manion L, Morrison K. *Research Methods in Education.* 8th ed. London and New York: Routledge; 2018.
9. Mason J. *Qualitative Researching.* London: Sage; 1996.
10. Burgess RG. *In the Field: An Introduction to Field Research.* London: Unwin Hyman; 1984.
11. Schwandt TA. *Dictionary of Qualitative Inquiry.* 2nd ed. Thousand Oaks, CA: Sage; 2001.
12. Block ES, Erskine L. Interviewing by telephone: specific considerations, opportunities, and challenges. *Int J Qual Methods* 2012;11(4):428–445.

13. Salmons J. *Qualitative Online Interviews*. 2nd ed. Thousand Oaks: Sage; 2015.

14. Krueger RA, Casey MA. *Focus Groups: A Practical Guide for Applied Research*. 5th ed. Thousand Oaks: Sage; 2014.

15. Mack N, Woodsong C, MacQueen KM, Guest G, Namey E. *Qualitative Research Methods: A Data Collector's Field Guide*. Research Triangle Park, NC: Family Health International; 2005.

16. Gold RL. Roles in sociological field observations. *Soc Forces* 1958;36(3):217–223.

17. Green J, Thorogood N. *Qualitative Methods for Health Research*. 3rd ed. Los Angeles, CA: Sage; 2014.

18. Lincoln YS, Guba EG. *Naturalistic Inquiry*. Newbury Park, CA: Sage; 1985.

19. Bowen G. Document analysis as a qualitative research method. *Qual Res J* 2009;9(2):27–40.

20. Flick U. *The SAGE Handbook of Qualitative Data*. Los Angeles, CA: Sage; 2013.

21. Miles MB, Huberman AM. *Qualitative Data Analysis: An Expanded Sourcebook*. Thousand Oaks, CA: Sage; 1994.

22. Hsieh HF, Shannon SE. Three approaches to qualitative content analysis. *Qual Health Res* 2005;15(9):1277–1288.

23. Braun V, Clarke V. Using thematic analysis in psychology. *Qual Res Psychol* 2006;3(2):77–101.

CHAPTER 20

Action research

John Sandars

INTRODUCTION

Many primary care education researchers may not be familiar with action research,[1] although it has been widely used in other areas of education for over 50 years. Action research combines implementing a change in educational practice (the action component of action research) with greater understanding of the various factors that enable and constrain the change (the research component of action research). The potential usefulness of the findings from action research depends on the process of conducting the research, including the quality of data collection and analysis.

WHAT IS ACTION RESEARCH?

Implementation of a change in educational practice, such as a new approach to teaching or a new module in a curriculum, is a complex process and often the intended outcome may not be fully achieved, or there are unexpected outcomes. The process of implementation depends on a wide range of different inter-related factors that enable or constrain the change. There are important factors related to the design of the new practice. For example, effective implementation of an e-learning intervention requires the close alignment of the needs of the learner, the content, the instructional design, the technology and the context. However, there are additional important factors that are specifically related to the implementation within a particular context, such as the organisational culture and available resources. Identification and understanding of the factors can be used to modify further implementation of the change, but this may require several attempts for the intended outcome to be achieved. This iterative process with cycles of implementation (action) and increased understanding (research) is an essential feature of action research.

There are two main types of action research: individual and participatory. Individual action research has a focus on improving the educational practice of only one educator but sometimes there can be collaboration between several educators. This type of action research has been mainly used for faculty and staff development.

Participatory action research has been more widely used for implementing change in educational practice and there is active participation of a range of different stakeholders, such as learners and administrators, in all phases of the implementation and research.

The term 'research' is used in action research since there is an enquiry into an event (the implementation), and appropriate research methods, such as qualitative research with focus groups, are used to collect and analyse information about the implementation. However, a key aspect of action research is critical reflection. For individual type of action research, this reflection usually has a focus on developing the personal and professional self-awareness which is essential for improving professional practice. For the participatory type of action research, reflection has a greater focus on the important organisational factors, including the power dynamics between the various stakeholders involved in the implementation.

HOW TO PERFORM ACTION RESEARCH?

Action research has several phases and usually more than one cycle:

Cycle One

Phases

1. Identification of a problem with current educational practice
2. Research the problem by initial data collection and analysis
3. Develop a proposed solution to the problem
4. Implement the proposed solution to the problem
5. Research the implementation of the solution by data collection and analysis
6. Identify the factors that enable and constrain the implementation of the solution which may also include factors that are in the proposed solution
7. Develop a modified proposed solution based on the identified factors
8. Implement the modified proposed solution
9. Research the implementation of the solution by data collection and analysis

Critical reflection occurs in Phases 5, 6 and 7.

Cycle Two

All of the phases in Cycle Two are repeated until the problem with current educational practice has been resolved.

More details of the process of action research are available in the 'Recommended Reading' section, as are two illustrative examples. The first example is a group of clinical educators and a new clinical reasoning course, and the second is a participatory project with the local community and a new curriculum for ensuring that it was responsive to the needs of persons in poverty.

Many action research projects are limited to only Cycle One, especially when there are time constraints. However, for both individual and participatory action research, the intended potential benefits of obtaining greater understanding are likely to be reduced if there are no cycles of critical reflection. See section 'Recommended Reading' for an illustrative example of action research using several cycles to implement training about obesity management.

The use of qualitative and quantitative research methods should follow recommended guidance on data collection and analysis to ensure that appropriate validity and reliability are achieved. This is essential if action research is to be more widely disseminated, especially for submission for publication.

Action research is similar to educational design research which also has several phases within iterative cycles. An illustrative example of an educational design research project and an innovative approach for feedback in clinical settings is provided in section 'Recommended Reading'.

THE STRENGTHS AND LIMITATIONS OF ACTION RESEARCH

The main strength of action research is that it combines implementation of a change and greater understanding within a specific real-life context. However, there are several limitations of action research. A major limitation is often the time required to conduct several cycles and the lack of familiarity of the overall process of action research. There are often concerns about generalisability, but the findings from action research can inform the design and implementation of new interventions in other contexts by identifying major themes.

CONCLUSION

Action research plays an important role in primary care education research by combining implementation and greater understanding. The development of greater understanding about both the individual, with increased self-awareness, and the context, with the complexity of different factors in an organisation, is an essential aspect of action research.

RECOMMENDED READING

Methodology of action research
Open access

O'Brien, R. (2001). Um exame da abordagem metodológica da pesquisa ação [An overview of the methodological approach of action research]. In: Roberto Richardson, ed. *Teoria e Prática da Pesquisa Ação [Theory and Practice of Action Research]*. João Pessoa, Brazil: Universidade Federal da Paraíba. (English version) Available from: http://www.web.ca/~robrien/papers/arfinal.html (Accessed 10 September 2020).

Publications

Chen W, Reeves TC. Twelve tips for conducting educational design research in medical education. *Med Teach* 2019;42(9): 980–986. doi:10.1080/0142159X.2019.1657231

Coghlan D. *Doing Action Research in Your Own Organization.* 5th ed. Sage; London, UK. 2019.

McKenney S, Reeves TC. *Conducting Educational Design Research.* 2nd ed. Routledge;London, UK 2018.

McNiff J. *You and Your Action Research Project.* 4th ed. Routledge; London, UK 2016.

Illustrative examples of action research
Open access

Delany C, Golding C. Teaching clinical reasoning by making thinking visible: an action research project with allied health clinical educators. *BMC Med Educ* 2014;14:20. doi:10.1186/1472-6920-14-20

Hudon C, Loignon C, Grabovschi C, et al. Medical education for equity in health: a participatory action research involving persons living in poverty and healthcare professionals. *BMC Med Educ* 2016;6:106. doi:10.1186/s12909-016-0630-4

Publication

Leedham-Green KE, Pound R, Wylie A. Enabling tomorrow's doctors to address obesity in a GP consultation: an action research project. *Educ Prim Care* 2016;27(6):455–61. doi:10.1080/14739879.2016.1205459

Illustrative example of educational design research
Open access

Leggett HD. (2016). Helping Clinical Educators Provide Effective Feedback to Medical Trainees on Their Diagnostic Decision Making: An Educational Design Research Approach. PhD thesis, University of Leeds. Available from: http://etheses.whiterose.ac.uk/id/eprint/13434 (Accessed 10 September 2020).

REFERENCE

1. Sandars J, Singh G, McPherson M. Are we missing the potential of action research for transformative change in medical education? *Educ Prim Care* 2012;23(4):239–241. doi: 10.1080/14739879.2012.11494115

CHAPTER 21

Case study research

John Sandars

INTRODUCTION

While many medical education researchers are not familiar with case study research, it has been used for over 2,000 years to obtain greater understanding of clinical problems and concerns. An early example is Herodotus, who lived in Ancient Greece, and his quest to better understand the triggers of suicide in soldiers.[1] He identified the various contributory factors in each of the nine cases that he studied, and then compared the factors from across the cases. This inquiry-led approach has been widely applied in education research,[2] and is highly applicable to primary care medical education research.

WHAT IS CASE STUDY RESEARCH?

Case study research has a focus on a specific case to obtain an in-depth understanding of a problem or concern that is present within a particular context. The case and the context have to be clearly defined from the outset of the research, and the choice will depend on the research question. For example, a researcher may be interested in why students on a specific inner-city primary care placement are not experiencing the health care provided to homeless families. The case in this example is 'the specific inner-city primary care placement in which there is a problem'. If the researcher is interested in all of the inner-city primary care placements that are provided by the medical school, the case is 'all of these placements within the specific context of the medical school'. It is important to clearly state the case that is being studied, since the results obtained from the research are only directly related to this case.

A key aspect of case study research is the in-depth understanding of what and/or why something is occurring in the case. Exploratory qualitative research methods are an essential component of case study research, and the additional use of quantitative methods as a mixed methods research approach can provide greater in-depth understanding.

Case study research can be combined with other research studies, such as a questionnaire survey, to provide in-depth understanding of what is being studied. The choice of cases should be purposive, with an intention to obtain cases that can provide a unique perspective. Using the previous example of primary care placements, the choice of cases could be the placements that are at the extremes of the sample. These cases would be the placements in which students had a very high experience compared with the extreme of very low experience.

HOW TO PERFORM CASE STUDY RESEARCH?

Similar to all research, there has to be a clear and specific research question. The choice of case tends to be the most challenging aspect of performing case study research, and the reader is advised to consult the articles in the recommended reading before commencing the research. The use of qualitative and quantitative research methods should follow recommended guidance on data collection and analysis to ensure that appropriate validity and reliability are achieved.

THE STRENGTHS AND LIMITATIONS OF CASE STUDY RESEARCH

The main strength of case study research is the in-depth understanding within a specific context. For example, several important themes were identified in a case study of the experience of the lead educator in establishing new multi-disciplinary training centres in the specific North West region of the United Kingdom.[3] Although only five interviews were performed, the data collected had a large amount of detail, and the major themes were consistent across all of the leads. These themes included their motivation and expectations for the training centres, the benefits that were achieved by learners and practice staff, the challenges of implementation and the barriers to sustainability.

The main limitation of most case study research is the extent to which the findings are only based on a specific case within a particular context. This concern about generalisability, which is the extent to which the research findings from one study can be applied to other settings, is frequently highlighted by other researchers and reviewers of journal articles. These concerns can be overcome by presenting the findings as an instrumental rather than an intrinsic case study.[4] An intrinsic case study only explores a single case, but an instrumental case study provides greater understanding of a problem or concern with wider implications that can be applied to other settings. In the previous example of training centres, the case study was instrumental, and identified factors to be considered for wider implementation, including the support networks for the lead educators, adequate funding, maintaining good communication between the lead educators and the policymakers and the careful management of the number of learners.

Greater applicability of the findings of case study research can be achieved by using multiple case studies, such as across different countries, and performing cross-case synthesis and analysis to identify themes that are common across all of the studies.

The lack of sufficient rigour in the collection and analysis of data in case study research also increases the legitimate concerns about the limitations of the findings. It is essential to follow the recommended guidance on data collection and analysis for the qualitative, quantitative and mixed methods approaches being used.

CONCLUSION

Case study research has an important place in primary care education research by providing in-depth understanding of a problem or concern. Illustrative examples related to medical education are provided in the recommended reading. It is essential that the whole process, from selection of cases to data collection and analysis, is clearly described and conforms to recommended guidance. The recommended reading provides useful articles on the methodology of case study research. Finally, to ensure that the findings from case study approach are applicable to other settings, it is important to identify themes that can inform wider understanding of a problem or concern.

RECOMMENDED READING – OPEN ACCESS RESOURCES

Methodology of case study research

Crowe S, Cresswell K, Robertson A, Huby G, Avery A, Sheikh A. The case study approach. *BMC Med Res Method* 2011 Dec;11(1):100. doi:10.1186/1471-2288-11-100

Fàbregues S, Fetters MD. Fundamentals of case study research in family medicine and community health. *Fam Med Comm Health* 2019 Mar 1;7(2):e000074. Available from: https://fmch.bmj.com/content/7/2/e000074

Illustrative examples of case study research

Lemos AR, Sandars JE, Alves P, Costa MJ. The evaluation of student-centredness of teaching and learning: a new mixed-methods approach. *Int J Med Educ* 2014;5:157. doi:10.5116/ijme.53cb.8f87

O'Callaghan C, Sandars J, Brown J, Sherratt C. The use of mixed methods social network analysis to evaluate healthcare professionals' educator development: an exploratory study. *J Contemp Med Educ* 2020;10(1):15–26. doi:10.5455/jcme.20191120122732

Yeung S, Bombay A, Walker C, et al. Predictors of medical student interest in Indigenous health learning and clinical practice: a Canadian case study. *BMC Med Educ* 2018 Dec 1;18(1):307. doi:10.1186/s12909-018-1401-1

REFERENCES

1. Pridmore S, Auchincloss S, Ahmadi J. Suicide triggers described by Herodotus. *Iran J Psychiatry.* 2016: 11(2):128–132. magiran.com/p1543825
2. Brown PA. A review of the literature on case study research. *Can J New Schol Educ* 2008;1(1):1–13. Available from: https://jmss.org/index.php/cjnse/article/view/30395
3. Brown JM, Sandars JE, Nwolise C, et al. Multi-disciplinary training hubs in North West England: the training hub lead perspective. *Educ Prim Care* 2019 Sep 3;30(5):289–294. doi:10.1080/14739879.2019.1639553
4. Stake RE. Case studies (Chapter 16). In: Denzin NK, Lincoln YS, eds. *Handbook of Qualitative Research.* Thousand Oaks, CA: Sage; 2000: 435–454.

CHAPTER 22

Individual interviews and focus groups

Kathryn Hoffmann

BACKGROUND

Medical education is a complex field which synthesises multiple perspectives, intentions and motivations on how students learn and how medicine should be taught.[1-3] One of the tools for research is interviewing, either one-on-one or more than one person at a time, in focus groups.[4]

ONE-ON-ONE INTERVIEWS

One-on-one interviews can be either semi-structured or in-depth. The former *are conducted on the basis of a loose structure of open questions* [interview guideline], *which define the area to be explored, at least initially, and from which the interviewer or interviewee may diverge in order to pursue an idea in more detail.*[5] In-depth interviews *are less structured than this, and may cover only one or two issues, but in great detail.*[5] For both, the aim is to go below the surface and uncover perspectives and beliefs unknown prior to the start of the research,[5] to motivate interviewees to explain and describe their own beliefs and understandings in as much detail as possible in their own words.[5-7]

Common pitfalls in interviewing include interruptions from outside, competing distractions, stage-fright for interviewer or interviewee, asking embarrassing or awkward questions, jumping from one subject to another, teaching instead of interviewing (e.g. giving the interviewee medical advice), counselling instead of interviewing (e.g. summarising responses too early), presenting one's own perspective and superficial interviews.[6]

An example of a semi-structured interview study in medical education is a French study about medical errors by trainee general practitioners, a very sensitive topic.[8] Interviewees have to be chosen with respect to the research question, and to fit the particular profile.[9] This is important because the way of explaining a phenomenon may vary, for example, according to the cultural significance of the topic, peer group interpretations and religious constructs.[10] Moreover, a person can be engaged in various levels of culture applying to a country, community or virtual group.[10] In general, the adequate number of interviews is reached when new interviews by the purposely selected participants give no further insights into the topic (data saturation).

While it is often said that sensitive topics should mainly be researched via one-on-one interviews,[4,6,11,12] a study from North Carolina found that *several types of sensitive and personal disclosures were more likely in a focus group setting, and that some sensitive themes only occurred in the focus group context. No sensitive themes emerged exclusively, or more often in, an individual interview context.*[13] This could lead to the speculation that it depends more on the type of people in the group and the performance of the interviewer, rather than on the kind of interview form. Nevertheless, to explore very sensitive, embarrassing or 'personal' topics, such as medical errors or sexual or racist harassment in the classroom, might still require individual interviews. Participants might not be comfortable in discussing these issues in front of other people, or the discussion might lead to emotional distress.[14] It is advantageous to consider strategies to support interviewees who become distressed by the interview, such as referral options to a helpline or care services. In any case, qualitative studies have to be approved by the ethics committee in advance.

FOCUS GROUPS

Focus groups typically consist of 6–10 (sometimes up to 12) participants plus the interviewer. With larger groups, it may be helpful to also have a group facilitator to run the recording and take notes.[5,15] Due to group dynamic issues, focus groups are in general more structured, and the interviewer follows an interview guideline to keep to the topic of interest. *Focus groups are structured around a set of carefully predetermined questions – usually no more than 10 – but the discussion is free-flowing. Ideally, participant comments will stimulate and influence the thinking and sharing of others. Some people even find themselves changing their thoughts and opinions during the group.*[15]

The main characteristic of a focus group is the interaction between the moderator and the group, as well as between group members.[12] Participants can either be homogeneous (share key features) or heterogeneous, with different characteristics, depending on the aim of the group regarding the topic (e.g. to challenge an idea, identify crucial points, explore interpersonal and rhetorical processes and social interaction or generate high consensus).[12,16]

In general, results of focus groups show cover breadth of the topic more than one-on-one interviews, where single answers are more in-depth.[4,5,7,16] However, to really be able to assess the breadth of the topic via focus groups, it usually takes more than one group to produce valid results. As with interviews, sufficient groups need to have been conducted with the same set of questions with no new material emerging.[12,15]

In a British example using focus groups, patients were asked about their views on student doctors in their general practice (GP) offices. The results showed important aspects to consider when organising GP-based teaching.[17] *Patients' enablement and satisfaction are not impaired by students' participation in consultations. Patients generally support the teaching of student doctors in their general practice but expect to be provided with sufficient information and to have a choice about participation, so they can give informed consent.*[17]

It should be noted that a focus group is not a debate, group therapy, conflict resolution session, problem-solving session, opportunity to collaborate, promotional opportunity, nor an educational session.[15] The interviewer role is of main importance – they must be able to deal with group dynamics, maintain the structure and the process of the focus group, include all participants equally, establish a climate of confidence and keep their personal views out.[5,7,12,15,18]

CONCLUSION

For the advantages and disadvantages of one-on-one interviews and focus groups, see Table 22.1. For both interview types, the role of the interviewer is key. If the interviewer is a physician, he or she must be aware that the interviewer role is profoundly different from that of a doctor. *Whereas the doctor is seeking to translate what the patient says [in the consultation] into the concepts which make up his/her own model, the qualitative researcher is concerned to understand, as fully as possible, the interviewee's concepts, rather than simply to translate them.*[5] This is similarly the case where a teacher is an interviewer. Where there is such a power imbalance, and interviewers represent persons of high social and societal ranking, care must be taken to avoid the 'please the interviewer' effect.[14]

TABLE 22.1 Summary of the advantages and disadvantages of interview types

	Advantages	Disadvantages
One-on-one interview	• In-depth analysis due to longer speaking time • Higher potential for deep insights, uncover perspectives and beliefs, unknown prior to the research • Helpful when participants are dispersed geographically or regarding their time schedule • Talk to only one person at a time • No worry about group dynamics that inevitably occur in focus groups • Interviewer can give interviewee full attention and adjust interviewing style to meet interviewee's needs • Good in confidential situations	• Organisation of many interviews • May be more complex to interpret • Artificial interviewing situation • Stronger 'please the interviewer effect' • No insight into social interactions regarding the topic • Pitfalls include external interruptions, competing distractions, 'stage-fright', embarrassing or awkward questions, jumping from one subject to another, teaching or counselling instead of interviewing, presenting own perspective, superficial interviews
Focus group	• Diversity of interviewees' profiles and enrichment of responses • Explore breadth of a topic • Explore interpersonal and rhetorical processes and social interaction on a topic • Simulate more real-world responses • Observe commonalities and differences between participants	• Speaking time of attendees may be unequal • Lower average speaking time of all participants • Moderator's bias hard to prevent • May be difficult to organise when potential participants live in different regions or have different time schedules • Social and group dynamics can bias the results • Safeguarding and confidentiality issues

REFERENCES

1. Albert M, Hodges B, Regehr G. Research in medical education: balancing service and science. *Adv Health Sci Educ* 2007;12(1):103–115. doi:10.1007/s10459-006-9026-2
2. Cristancho S, Varpio L. Twelve tips for early career medical educators. *Med Teach* 2016;38(4):358–363. doi:10.3109/0142159X.2015.1062084
3. Sawatsky AP, Ratelle JT, Beckman TJ. Qualitative research methods in medical education. *Anesthesiology* 2019;131(1):14–22. doi:10.1097/aln.0000000000002728
4. Zaharia RM. Qualitative research methods: a comparison between focus-group and in-depth interview. *Ann Fac Econ* 2008;4(1):1279–1283.
5. Britten N, Jones R, Murphy E, et al. Qualitative research methods in general practice and primary care. *Fam Pract* 1995;12(1):104–114. doi:10.1093/fampra/12.1.104
6. Britten N. Qualitative interviews in medical research. *BMJ* 1995;311(6999):251–253. doi:10.1136/bmj.311.6999.251
7. Flick U. *Qualitative Sozialforschung. Eine Einführung.* Hamburg: Rowohlt Taschenbuch Verlag; 2016.
8. Venus E, Galam E, Aubert J-P, et al. Medical errors reported by French general practitioners in training: results of a survey and individual interviews. *BMJ Qual Safety* 2012;21(4):279–286. doi:10.1136/bmjqs-2011-000359
9. Sofaer S. Qualitative research methods. *Int J Qual Health Care* 2002;14(4):329–336. doi:10.1093/intqhc/14.4.329
10. Hammarberg K, Kirkman M, de Lacey S. Qualitative research methods: when to use them and how to judge them. *Hum Reprod* 2016;31(3):498–501. doi:10.1093/humrep/dev334
11. Wong L. Qualitative research methods in family medicine: what and why? *Malays Fam Physician* 2008;3(1):70.
12. Wong LP. Focus group discussion: a tool for health and medical research. *Singapore Med J* 2008;49(3):256–260.
13. Guest G, Namey E, Taylor J, et al. Comparing focus groups and individual interviews: findings from a randomized study. *Int J Soc Res Methodol* 2017;20(6):693–708.
14. Maheshwari. Focus Groups vs. One-on-One Interviews (When and Why): UXArmy – online user testing platform; 2019. Available from: https://medium.com/uxarmy/focus-groups-vs-one-on-one-interviews-when-and-why-9ad38ee16ef5.
15. Associates E. Guidelines for Conducting a Focus Group: The University of Mississippi, Office of Institutional Research, Effectiveness, and Planning; 2005. Available from: https://irep.olemiss.edu/wp-content/uploads/sites/98/2016/05/Trinity_Duke_How_to_Conduct_a_Focus_Group.pdf.
16. James A. Planning and conducting interviews and focus groups; 2017. Available from: https://www.srhe.ac.uk/downloads/events/301_alanajames.pdf.
17. Benson J, Quince T, Hibble A, et al. Impact on patients of expanded, general practice based, student teaching: observational and qualitative study. *BMJ* 2005;331(7508):89. doi:10.1136/bmj.38492.599606.8F
18. Krueger RA. Designing and Conducting Focus Group Interviews: University of Minesota; 2002. Available from: https://www.eiu.edu/ihec/Krueger-FocusGroupInterviews.pdf

CHAPTER 23

Content analysis: a guide for primary health care education researchers

Kyle Eggleton

BACKGROUND

Content analysis is a data analysis method that aims to reduce data down into smaller categories in order to gain some form of deeper insight. The intention of qualitative content analysis methods is to generate a broad description of data in order to develop or prove a theory.[1] The aim of this chapter is to understand qualitative content analysis through the use of examples and apply this method to primary health care education research. The context of the example study is interviews of student community health workers (CHW) who have undertaken a period of training with a CHW in a small village. The aim of this example study is to ascertain how students understand the role of a CHW.

TYPES OF CONTENT ANALYSIS

There are two broad approaches to qualitative content analysis and these are based on deductive or inductive methods. Inductive content analysis (also known as conventional content analysis[2]) involves a 'ground-up' analysis of the data that attempts to reflect the experiences or meaning of the owners of the text. On the other hand, deductive content analysis uses pre-existing theory to analyse data. In addition, two depths of analysis can occur – either manifest or latent analysis (Box 23.1). Within manifest analysis, words are taken at their face value or original meaning. In contrast, latent analysis is

---

BOX 23.1   MANIFEST VERSUS LATENT ANALYSIS

In the following quote, a student CHW is asked what they do to ensure that patients are well.

> I would go into homes with the community health worker and ask if anyone is unwell. Often people might have a fever and I would check their pulse...

A manifest analysis code, applied to this text, might be *checking for illness*. However, in latent analysis, the pause at the end of the sentence and the lack of referral to the primary health care nurse might reflect uncertainty around dealing with illnesses and an appropriate code might be *uncertainty with illnesses*.

---

meaning of the underlying text or the hidden meaning.[3] With latent content analysis, non-verbals or utterances are also noted.

UNDERTAKING AN ANALYSIS
Determining the source of data

The source of data for content analysis varies, but can include other papers, such as undertaking a literature review of papers reporting on trends in distance education[4]; media reports, such as exploring the use of Twitter in medical education[5]; written material, such as analysing online discussion forums of medical students[6] or analysing nursing school curricula[7]; of interviews, for example, exploring the experiences of student-run clinics in primary care[8] and personal journals, such as analysing reflective logs of medical students.[9]

PREPARING FOR CODING

Once the source of date is determined, the next step is deciding on the unit of analysis, generally a whole interview or a discrete collection of data. Following this, the meaning unit is clarified, i.e. words, sentences or paragraphs that relate to each other.

BOX 23.2   UNIT OF ANALYSIS AND MEANING UNITS

In the study of student CHWs, the researcher decides to use individual interviews with each student as the unit of analysis and one to two sentences as the meaning unit that they will code.

After determining the size of the meaning units, codes are then applied to them. A variety of different software programmes exist to assist in this process; however, there are also valid manual approaches. For example, researchers could use a spreadsheet and copy and paste data into individual cells, then attribute a code to that meaning unit in an adjacent cell.

Inductive coding

There are a number of different steps involved in inductive content analysis.

1. *Decontextualisation* is the process of breaking the data down into smaller, more manageable chunks. The text is read and re-read and descriptive labels applied to meaning units to capture the underling meaning (whether that is manifest or latent).

BOX 23.3   APPLYING CODES IN INDUCTIVE CONTENT ANALYSIS

In the below example of decontextualisation, the researcher has copied and pasted text from the transcribed interviews into a spreadsheet and assigned codes to the meaning units

Transcribed Interview	Code
I guess one thing that I have found, with working with the community health worker for this village, is ummm, that the elderly people know them because they know their parents and can remember them I they were born, and that means that they trust her.	Trust from belonging
But, I think, umm, that people also trust the community health worker because she looks out for them and is fighting to get the right medicine and, you know, health care that they need	Trust due to positive action

---

2. *Recontextualisation* involves ensuring that the content is covered by the aim and that any uncoded text is not relevant. This involves re-reading the data and applying further codes if necessary.
3. *Categorisation* is the process through which themes or categories are developed, along with sub-categories or sub-headings. This involves reading through the various codes and grouping them into natural groupings. In the example above, the researcher decided to group

the codes of *trust from belonging* and *trust due to positive action* into one category called *building trust*. Category names should be self-explanatory and a definition built up of their meanings. Initial categories are often reduced in number through a process of abstraction into broader categories or themes. The term category and theme are often interchangeable; however, category tends to be used for manifest coding and theme for latent coding.

BOX 23.4   ABSTRACTION

Initial categories of the student CHW study include:

- Building trust
- Working alongside the community
- Getting buy-in

The researchers decide that these categories all relate to community development processes and so they create a new category encompassing them all.

Deductive coding

Deductive content analysis (also known as directed content analysis[2]) involves the initial creation of a categorisation matrix that defines and describes categories of data. The data are then coded according to this matrix, and finally all of the data are reviewed to determine if they exemplify the categories.[1]

BOX 23.5   CATEGORISATION MATRIX

Using a deductive approach, the researcher decided to create a categorisation matrix based on the social-ecological model. Four categories were created:

- Individual-level activity
- Interpersonal-level activity
- Organisational-level activity
- Environmental-level activity

The researcher then coded all of the interviews based on these categories to determine whether students' understanding of the roles and activities of CHWs was consistent with the social-ecological model.

Two subtypes of deductive content analysis exist, depending on the decision made at the beginning of the study on what to do with data that do not fit within the initial categorisation matrix. The first variation involves including only content that fits the matrix, to prove whether the theory holds or not. This type of deductive content analysis uses a constrained categorisation matrix.[1] With an unconstrained categorisation matrix, the text is coded with the categorisation matrix and then inductive coding is applied to the text not otherwise coded. Sometimes counts of categories or rank order of categories can occur in deductive content analysis. An example is the categorisation and counting of documented competencies recorded by family medicine residents.[10]

MAINTAINING TRUSTWORTHINESS

Trustworthiness of content analysis depends on a number of elements[11]:

- *Credibility*: How well the data address the aims.
- *Dependability*: Principles and criteria used for selecting data/ participants are clearly stated so that how the study might translate to other settings can be seen.
- *Conformability*: Data represent the information provided by the participants and that the results are not heavily dependent on the researcher.

Trustworthiness is increased by careful explanation of how the categories were created as well as detailed descriptions of the analysis process and through use of figures (such as a hierarchy of concepts and categories) and tables. In a deductive approach, double-coding assesses how good the categorisation matrix is. In an inductive approach, multiple researchers might check coding and discuss divergent opinion.

CONCLUSION

There are a number of caveats with content analysis. For example, deductive content analysis may result in more supportive evidence being found, rather than un-supportive evidence, due to pre-existing bias of the researchers with their knowledge of the theory used.[2] For inductive content analysis, there are often limitations in theory development, compared to say grounded theory, due to issues around sampling and analysis processes.[2] Despite these caveats, content analysis provides a useful and approachable method for primary health care education researchers in analysing a wide range of texts.

REFERENCES

1. Elo S, Kyngäs H. The qualitative content analysis process. *J Adv Nurs* 2008;62(1):107–115.
2. Hsieh H, Shannon S. Three approaches to qualitative content analysis. *Qual Health Res* 2005;15(9):1277–1288.

3. Bengtsson M. How to plan and perform a qualitative study using content analysis. *NursingPlus Open* 2016;2:8–14.

4. Bozkurt A, Akgun-Ozbek E, Yilmazel S, et al. Trends in distance education research: a content analysis of journals 2009-2013. *Int Rev Res Open Dis Learn* 2015;16(1):330–363.

5. Jalali A, Sherbino J, Frank J, Sutherland S. Social media and medical education: exploring the potential of Twitter as a learning tool. *Int Rev Psychiatry* 2015;27(2):140–146.

6. Gillingham K, Eggleton K, Goodyear-Smith F. Is reflective learning visible in online discussion forums for medical students on general practice placements? A qualitative study. *Teach Learn Med* 2020;1–8.

7. Aase I, Aase K, Dieckmann P. Teaching interprofessional teamwork in medical and nursing education in Norway: a content analysis. *J Interprof Care* 2013;27(3):238–245.

8. Fröberg M, Leanderson C, Fläckman B, et al. Experiences of a student-run clinic in primary care: a mixed-method study with students, patients and supervisors. *Scand J Prim Health Care* 2018;36(1):36–46.

9. Niemi PM. Medical students' professional identity: self-reflection during the preclinical years. *Med Educ* 1997;31(6):408–415.

10. Page C, Reid A, Brown M, Baker H, Coe C, Myerholtz L. Content analysis of family medicine resident peer observations. *Fam Med* 2020;52(1):43–47.

11. Elo S, Kääriäinen M, Kanste O, Pölkki T, Utriainen K, Kyngäs H. Qualitative content analysis: a focus on trustworthiness. *SAGE Open* 2014;4(1):1–10.

CHAPTER 24

Ethnography

Alex Harding

DEFINITION

Ethnography is a form of qualitative research where researchers observe the subject matter by immersing themselves in it – often for extended periods of time. Unlike more objective forms of research, it involves the researcher participating in the setting or interacting with the people being studied.

SHORT HISTORY

Originally ethnography started out in anthropology; observing and participating in other cultures – often over many years – to gain insights into our own cultures. However, today ethnography is far more diverse – other cultures, our own cultures, short immersion and prolonged immersion are all perfectly acceptable. However, the ethnographer is always to some extent a 'visitor'. Many ethnographic accounts, therefore, have a beguiling flavour to them, demonstrating deep knowledge of the subject – yet at the same time appearing to observe from afar.

HOW TO DO ETHNOGRAPHY?

Make sure that ethnography is the best method to answer your research question. Plan early. Have an idea of what you are looking for before you start. Getting ethical approval to do ethnography can be difficult and time-consuming. In addition, gaining permission from the subject (often a health care provider) to observe medical practice (which is different to ethical approval) can also prove difficult. Periods of a year or more are not uncommon.

What are your motives for doing this work? Be honest. What might prejudice your observations? In short, be 'reflexive' – aware of how your prejudices and motives for doing the work might affect your observations and conclusions.

Plan the outline structure of your ethnography:

a. These days, it's fine to do 'focussed' ethnography.[1] This significantly reduces the amount of time spent observing, but you need to have a good idea of what it is you want to observe.
b. What kind of observation do you want to do?
   i.   Participant observation: You join in with everything – the parties, induction rituals and more. Just think – how feasible is this?
   ii. Quasi-participant observation: The middle ground.
   iii. Non-participant observation: You don't really interact with those you are observing. Just think; how realistic is this?

It is really important to pilot the observations. When you actually start observations, there is often a sharp reality jolt. For example, in my work, I was focussing on the role of curriculum in shaping clinical learning. It became quickly apparent that curriculum played little part and so major adaptations were needed to the design.[2,3]

When you are ready, what do you 'do' when observing?

Firstly, wake up! look!, listen! smell! feel! – you are trying to be 'in' the world that your subject's inhabit. It is very hard and demanding work. Practising meditation – clearing your mind and focussing on the here and now – can be a useful preparation for observation.

Secondly, take lots of notes. However, sometimes you cannot take notes and you just observe, trying to remember as much as possible, but do not leave it too long. An A5-size notebook is ideal for notes, as it's not too intrusive, or a small laptop. A smartphone is indispensable – record off-the-cuff interviews, if possible and with consent, take photos – they can save a thousand words.

Remember that collecting 'artefacts' can be useful as well. Pieces of paper outlining 'official' codes, practices and rules are often useful to contrast with the reality of what is being observed.

You need to try hard, all of the time to integrate yourself – offering to buy coffee is an excellent ice breaker. A treat, a chance to top up caffeine levels to help you concentrate and a chance to talk to those you are observing. If you are invited to do things – do them – within reason.

ANALYSIS

This is often the 'weakest link' in qualitative work. Analysis takes place gradually (or 'iteratively'). After your first observations, return home to write up and think about what you have observed. Potential themes, questions, theories and explanations for what you have seen will spring up. These are what you check with your subjects the next time you do observations (checking and constant comparison).

Look for examples or people who do not conform to your emerging understanding (negative case analysis). Remember, you are aiming to describe in such a clear and detailed way to the reader that they can actually feel like they are there. Use sights, sounds, emotions to convey this.

As you gather data, look for 'patterns' or themes. You can use software to help this such as N-Vivo – but this is not obligatory. How are themes connected? Test your understanding in subsequent observations (more constant comparison). Try and get to the stage where coming in to observe produces relatively few things that you have not seen before (data saturation).

WRITING UP AND EXAMPLES OF GOOD ETHNOGRAPHY

Good ethnography is good communication. Discipline yourself to regular writing and rewriting. Drafting and redrafting is part of the craft. Read other people's work. There are plenty of good medical ethnographies.[4-7] However, these are mostly situated in hospitals, usually written in book form – it is difficult to distil ethnography into a paper, and this is worth bearing in mind before you start ethnography. The most famous ethnography is 'boys in white'.[5] The four authors spent two years during the early 1960s at an American medical school observing and performing interviews, but with very little preconceived ideas about what they might find. A more modern and focussed hospital ethnography is 'making doctors'[4] from a London school in the early 1990s. This ethnography uses a 'theoretical perspective' (a certain philosophical viewpoint) to focus observations, so is a little more focussed. However, perhaps the most fascinating is 'the body multiple' – an ethnography of Dutch vascular surgeons using the perspective of Actor-Network-Theory. While not easy to read, its presentation, the language used and the conclusions are fascinating.

With increasing amounts of time being spent by medical students in general practice, what is really needed now is an ethnography of education in general/family practice.

CONCLUSION

Ethnography is demanding and ethnographers inevitably 'get in the way' with what is being observed; you cannot observe something without changing it in some way, this is known as the Hawthorne effect.[8]

However, ethnography provides privileged and direct access to what is being studied. It is not like interviews or questionnaires that ask people what they think they do – it is observing what people and things actually do. The differences can be profound. Becker[5] spent eight years observing and interviewing medical students. The differences between what they said and what they did were so profound that his team discarded all interview data.

REFERENCES

1. Morris C. Reimagining 'the firm'; Clinical attachments as time spent in communities of practice. In: Cook V, Daly C, Newman M, eds. *Work-based Learning in Clinical Settings.* London: Radcliffe Publishing; 2012;17–20.
2. Harding AM. *How do medical students learn technical proficiency on hospital placements? The role of learning networks.* University College London; 2017.
3. Harding A. Actor-network-theory and micro-learning networks. *Educ Prim Care* 2017;28(5):295–296.
4. Sinclair S. *Making Doctors: An Institutional Apprenticeship.* Oxford: Oxford International Publishers Limited; 1997.
5. Becker HS, Geer B, Hughes EC, et al. *Boys in White: Student Culture in Medical School.* Chicago: The University of Chicago Press; 1961.
6. Atkinson P. *Medical Talk and Medical Work.* London: Sage; 1995.
7. Konner M. *Becoming a Doctor.* London: Penguin; 1987.
8. Parsons HM. What happened at Hawthorne? New evidence suggests the Hawthorne effect resulted from operant reinforcement contingencies. *Science* 1974;183(4128):922–932.

CHAPTER 25

Doing a mixed methods research or evaluation project

Michael D. Fetters

Astute clinicians routinely obtain a detailed history, make observations during the examination and use 'numbers' from testing to integrate clinical information about patients. As in clinical care, using stories and numbers can be used to address educational research challenges using mixed methods research (Box 25.1).

Mixed methods research is a cutting-edge methodology that uses an integrated approach for collecting qualitative and quantitative data.[2,3] Educational researchers can use mixed procedures to research teaching interventions or evaluate effectiveness of education strategies to achieve a holistic understanding that is greater than just a sum of the individual parts.[4]

BOX 25.1 CLINICAL EDUCATION STORY

You have been frustrated by your own and family medicine residents' lack of success with smoking cessation. You read an article about smoking cessation interventions where varenicline had the highest quit rate.[1] You decide to implement an educational intervention in your training program involving an intervention with the doctors in training to have them offer a varenicline prescription during all visits with smokers in your outpatient clinic. How can you show that your intervention works?

VARIATIONS IN DATA COLLECTION PROCEDURES

Some data collection procedures are inherently mixed, e.g. Delphi technique and mixed data collection surveys.[5] Analysis of secondary datasets or 'big' data are commonly quantitative, but can be qualitative or mixed. Field observations,[6] case study,[7] quality improvement,[8] curriculum development,[9] semi-structured interviews,[10] action research, ethnography, are commonly qualitative, but may be mixed. See other chapters also. Doing a mixed methods study requires collecting, analysing and integrating quantitative and qualitative data.[2,3] As many approaches can be used to research a specific topic, consider completing a methods-choosing exercise.[11] This chapter focuses on critical elements for conducting an integrated mixed methods study.

IDENTIFYING A TOPIC AND MIXED METHODS RESEARCH

Daily work in primary care raises numerous clinical and educational questions or dilemmas.[12] Such clinical stories, where you have doubts about optimal treatment or teaching strategies, or find conflicting literature about optimal choices, often lead to effective research topics.[11]

REVIEWING THE LITERATURE

In your literature review,[3] examine what kinds of projects have been done. How can these guide your project? If there is similar research, consider unique features of yours based on the setting or participants. For a mixed methods study, the literature review should justify collecting quantitative and qualitative data. Keep track of relevant literature for your write up.

MIXED METHODS RESEARCH QUESTIONS

Mixed methods research questions should include both a quantitative and qualitative component.[3] A mixed methods research question for the varenicline intervention (Box 25.1) could be *What are smoking patient quit rates and family medicine residents' experiences with routinely writing a varenicline prescription to smoking patients at every visit?* This research question illustrates the quantitative outcome – patient smoking cessation rates, and a qualitative assessment – residents' experiences in offering varenicline to smokers. As projects evolve, research questions invariably evolve too. When applying for research ethics committee approval, note that collecting quantitative and qualitative data can cause a greater participant burden, and render the informed consent process and protection of privacy more complex.

IDENTIFYING DATA SOURCES

When honing your research question, consider data sources available or feasible to collect for your research.[3] For the varenicline intervention

(Box 25.1), *quantitative data sources* could be 'quits' pre- to post-intervention, or pharmacy data quantifying the number of prescriptions filled. To confirm smoking cessation status, you could use a patient self-report measure, or check blood or saliva cotinine levels. *Qualitative data sources* could include text from patients' charts, semi-structured interviews[10] with resident physicians experienced in offering varenicline intervention to describe their level of enthusiasm and perception of patient receptivity. *Mixed data collection evaluations*, e.g. ratings based on scales from strongly agree to strongly disagree (Likert scale ratings), as well as written comments following a teaching conference about varenicline prescribing could be used.[5]

CHOOSING A MIXED METHODS RESEARCH DESIGN AND CREATING A PROCEDURAL DIAGRAM

Mixed methods researchers commonly use three core designs and depict their procedures using a procedural diagram.[3,13] Figure 25.1 provides a template to use for choosing among them and depicting your own research design.

An *explanatory sequential mixed methods design*[3,13] involves an initial quantitative assessment followed by a qualitative build on the initial quantitative findings, such that the qualitative data help explain the previously collected quantitative findings. In the varenicline study, an approach could be collecting pre- post-intervention outcomes data, and formulating questions based on the findings for subsequent interviews.

An *exploratory sequential mixed methods design*[3,13] involves first exploring a phenomenon of interest qualitatively, and then using the findings to guide building of the subsequent quantitative data collection tool. In the varenicline example, baseline interviews could be conducted prior to the intervention. This qualitative front work could be used to build the educational intervention and its evaluation by identifying outcomes the residents feel would be worth evaluating. For example, while a 'full quit' may be the initial plan, resident interviews might suggest that even short-term quitting, or 'mini-quit', might be a worthy outcome measure.

A *convergent mixed methods research design*[3,13] involves collecting both qualitative and quantitative data matched to address similar constructs. If a survey and interviews are being used, to some degree, the mixed data collection should be matched. This means collecting qualitative and quantitative data about specific constructs, e.g. cost, convenience, perceived efficacy. Matching data collection helps ensure the ability to integrate the mixed findings.

Additionally, there are various advanced mixed methods designs, too many to discuss.[3,13] One of these, mixed methods case study, is a particularly appropriate design for primary care educational research.[3,7]

Explanatory Sequential Mixed Methods Design

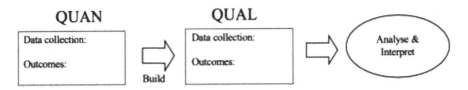

Exploratory Sequential Mixed Methods Design

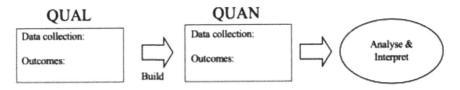

Convergent Mixed Methods Design

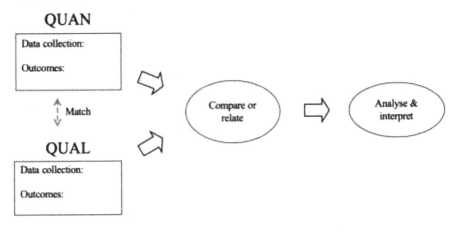

Instructions: 1) Choose from the three designs, 2) Record the data collection procedure you will use for the quantitative and qualitative data collection, 3) Record the outcomes you expect from both the quantitative and qualitative approaches

FIGURE 25.1 Three core mixed methods designs.

In such studies, researchers use a variety of available data sources and bound the case study, e.g. a varenicline case study could be bounded to family medicine residents in a single clinic, or residents and faculty from a multi-site training programme.

ANALYSING MIXED METHODS DATA

Data analysis for both quantitative[14] and qualitative data[15] should follow widely accepted steps and procedures. Mixed methods analysis[3] additionally includes: (1) conducting a data collection inventory, (2) framing the analysis according to your study questions, (3) describing patterns in your mixed data, (4) using an organisational structure for summarising findings,[16] (5) making interpretations by drawing interpretations based on both types of data (called meta-inferences), (6) organising results for dissemination and (7) interpreting the mixed findings and writing up the results.

CONCLUSION

While mixed methods projects encumber additional work, collecting and analysing both stories and numbers as in clinical work can be rewarding. An online special issue[17] and the *Mixed Methods Research Workbook*[3] are resources providing practical support for achieving the Box 25.2 checklist for conducting a mixed methods project.

BOX 25.2   CHECKLIST FOR CONDUCTING A MIXED METHODS STUDY

- Identify a relevant clinical education topic
- Review literature to support collection of quantitative and qualitative data
- Develop and refine iteratively a mixed methods research question
- Identify potential data sources to answer your mixed methods question
- Choose a relevant mixed methods research design
- Use an integrated strategy such that findings from one source can inform the other
- Collect and analyse each type of data
- Analyse and represent the data for publication using joint display techniques[17]

REFERENCES

1. Nides M, Glover ED, Reus VI, et al. Varenicline versus bupropion SR or placebo for smoking cessation: a pooled analysis. *Am J Health Behav* 2008;32(6):664–675.
2. Fetters MD, Curry LA, Creswell JW. Achieving integration in mixed methods designs-principles and practices. *Health Serv Res* 2013;48(6 Pt 2):2134–2156.
3. Fetters MD. *The Mixed Methods Research Workbook-Activities for Designing, Implementing, and Publishing Projects.* Thousand Oaks, CA: Sage Publications; 2020.

4. Fetters MD, Freshwater D. The 1 + 1 = 3 integration challenge. *JMMR* 2015;9(2):115–117.
5. Creswell JW, Hirose M. Mixed methods and survey research in family medicine and community health. *Fam Med Community Health* 2019;7(2):e000086.
6. Fetters MD, Rubinstein EB. The 3 Cs of content, context, and concepts: a practical approach to recording unstructured field observations. *Ann Fam Med* 2019;17(6):554–560.
7. Fabregues S, Fetters MD. Fundamentals of case study research in family medicine and community health. *Fam Med Community Health* 2019;7(2):e000074.
8. Ursu A, Greenberg G, McKee M. Continuous quality improvement methodology: a case study on multidisciplinary collaboration to improve chlamydia screening. *Fam Med Community Health* 2019;7(2):e000085.
9. Schneiderhan J, Guetterman TC, Dobson ML. Curriculum development: a how to primer. *Fam Med Community Health* 2019;7(2):e000046.
10. DeJonckheere M, Vaughn LM. Semistructured interviewing in primary care research: a balance of relationship and rigour. *Fam Med Community Health* 2019;7(2):e000057.
11. Fetters MD. Getting started in primary care research: choosing among six practical research approaches. *Fam Med Community Health* 2019;7(2):e000042.
12. Ventres W, Whiteside-Mansell L. Getting started in research, redefined: five questions for clinically focused physicians in family medicine. *Fam Med Community Health* 2019;7(2):e000017.
13. Creswell JW. *A Concise Introduction to Mixed Methods Research*. Thousand Oaks, CA: Sage Publications; 2014.
14. Guetterman TC. Basics of statistics for primary care research. *Fam Med Community Health* 2019;7(2):e000067
15. Babchuk WA. Fundamentals of qualitative analysis in family medicine. *Fam Med Community Health* 2019;7(2):e000040.
16. Guetterman TC, Fetters MD, Creswell JW. Integrating quantitative and qualitative results in health science mixed methods research through joint displays. *Ann Fam Med* 2015;13(6):554–561.
17. Fetters MD, Guetterman TC. Discovering and doing family medicine and community health research. *Fam Med Community Health* 2019;7(2):e000084.

CHAPTER 26

Applying methodologies to the curriculum: researching curriculum development and delivery

John Epling

INTRODUCTION

When undertaking educational research, there is the natural tendency to lead with an idea for a new *thing* to teach or a new *way* to teach something, then set about trying to prove that new idea or new method 'worked'. However, the outcomes studied in such research often default to such soft outcomes as: learners' 'comfort' with the material, their 'intention' to practice in a certain way, etc. This is a particular problem in primary care educational research, as the frequency of presentation of certain diseases, not to mention their outcomes, is diluted by the broad population of our panels, making it more difficult to achieve the rate of outcomes needed to show a difference. Fortunately, there is a wealth of potentially researchable questions in curriculum development and delivery that are important to study. The key to accessing these questions is planning the educational design and delivery carefully, so that researchable questions are evident at each step in the process. Instructional design is an educational discipline focussed on the systematic design and development of education and training to effectively change behaviour and achieve results. This chapter reviews some of the tools of instructional design – the use of a generic curriculum development model, the role of instructional objectives and two popular educational evaluation models – to exemplify the conduct a curriculum development project that lends itself more readily to educational research.

CURRICULUM DEVELOPMENT MODELS

In the field of instructional design, curriculum development models are used to structure and systematise curriculum development. There are many different types of models that suit different instructional circumstances or different evaluative needs.[1] A well-known generic curriculum development model that remains suitable to most purposes is known as ADDIE (Analysis, Design, Development, Implementation and Evaluation; see Table 26.1).[2] The ADDIE model began as a system developed for instruction in the US Air Force in the 1970s and has persisted as a simple yet robust framework for designing instruction. ADDIE is a simple and useful framework because it can scale from the individual teaching session all the way up to a course curriculum or training programme. The use of a model such as ADDIE encourages the educator to methodically consider each step in the curriculum development process and ensure that a decision about instructional strategy or a learner assessment method flows from the needs analysis and leads clearly to the next steps in the model.

While ADDIE began as a linear, 'waterfall' model, with one step following after the other, it soon evolved into a more holistic, iterative model with the evaluation component in the centre – touching all other steps in the process (see Figure 26.1).[2] This layout reinforces the concept that opportunities for evaluation exist throughout the ADDIE model. The most obvious are large-scale programme evaluations, both internal/formative (focussing on improving the design and development of the curriculum) and external/summative (targeting the learners, customers and stakeholders of the instruction to determine the success of the project).

TABLE 26.1 ADDIE curriculum development model[2]

	Step	Description
A	Analysis	Front-end needs assessment that may include baseline learner competencies and characteristics, broad goals for the instruction, gaps in performance that must be addressed, etc.
D	Design	Comprehensive design of the curriculum, including the objectives, instructional strategies and sequencing, learner assessments and messaging.
D	Development	Preparation of instructional materials and assessments, faculty development activities, resources required to conduct the curriculum, etc.
I	Implementation	Implementation of the curriculum – from introduction through final summative learner evaluation.
E	Evaluation	Educational programme evaluation of the planning, design and conduct of the curriculum.

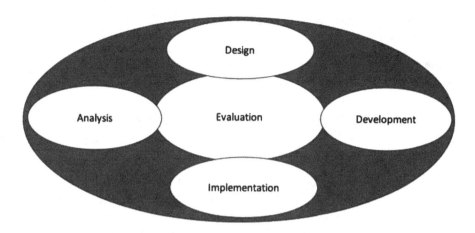

FIGURE 26.1 The ADDIE model with evaluation at its centre.

However, smaller-scale evaluations of each of the components of the model also can be useful. This broad range of potential evaluation topics can answer larger questions of whether the instruction met its intended goals in addition to more limited questions such as the adequacy of faculty and staff development, the performance and accuracy of assessment methods, the resources and time required to develop the instructional materials and the adequacy of the needs assessment process.

INSTRUCTIONAL OBJECTIVES

Writing clear and specific educational objectives is an integral part of the instructional design process. These objectives, when written properly, provide a clear description of the outcome desired as a result of the educational activity. Medical education has moved largely to competency-based learner assessment and has defined, for each level of education and specialty focus, the requisite assessable behaviours that are expected upon completion of their curricula. Behaviourally focussed educational objectives form the basis of a competency-based assessment scheme. A simple framework for writing specific educational objectives is 'ABCD' – audience, behaviour, condition, degree. The audience is the target for the educational intervention, the behaviour is observable change that is hoped for from the education, the conditions are any constraints or important context in which the behaviour is to be performed and degree is the extent to which the new behaviour is observed in order to qualify the education as a success.[3] For instance, an educational objective for teaching cardiac murmur identification in primary care might be: *The third-year resident (A) will be able to identify four common heart murmurs (B) when demonstrated on audiotape (C) with 100% success (D).*

TABLE 26.2 Mapping educational objectives (ABCD model) to educational PICOTS

Objectives	PICOTS
Audience	Population (learners)
Behaviour	Outcome
Condition	Timing, setting (possibly intervention)
Degree	Outcome definition, comparison

Educational objectives are specific about the outcome and level of achievement required of learners. It follows, then, that the educational researcher can use these objectives to plan the evaluation of the curriculum. A commonly used framework for developing research questions is the PICO(T)(S) model – patients/population, intervention, comparison, outcome (sometimes the timing and the setting of the study are included).[4] In the case of educational research, the 'patient/population' is usually the learners, since they are the ones undergoing the educational intervention. The ABCD model for writing objectives maps closely to the PICO(T)(S) model used to frame research questions, as seen in Table 26.2. Thoughtful development of the educational objectives, with the specificity offered by following a model such as ABCD, should lead directly into researchable questions for evaluating the curriculum.

The focus on educational objectives has come under some criticism for leading to an emphasis on what is easily measurable over what is an important educational outcome.[5,6] To counter this criticism, attention must be paid to the analysis portion of the ADDIE model, in which the important goals for the curriculum are learned, and the gaps between current and future practice are defined. Outcomes listed in the objectives should either match these goals, or, if accomplished, be relied upon to produce the larger goals.

EDUCATIONAL EVALUATION MODELS
As in the case of curriculum development models, there are several educational evaluation models that have gained wide acceptance. In the discussion of evaluation methods in education, it may be helpful to distinguish learner assessment (the degree to which the learner has accomplished the objectives of the educational activity as a result of the instruction) from the educational programme evaluation. This latter kind of evaluation is important for understanding the broader context, goals, feasibility and process of the educational activity.[7,8]

A well-known example of an evaluation model centred more around learner assessment is the Kirkpatrick Model of Training Evaluation (Table 26.3).[9,10] It was first published in 1994, and has been updated in recent years to refine

TABLE 26.3 'New World' Kirkpatrick training evaluation model[9,10]

Level	Description
Level 1 – Reaction	The degree to which the learners enjoyed the training and found it relevant
Level 2 – Knowledge	The degree to which the learners acquire new knowledge, skills, attitudes, confidence and commitment as a result of their training
Level 3 – Behaviour	The degree to which the learners' performance changes on the job as a result of the training
Level 4 – Results	The degree to which outcomes are affected by the training

and clarify it for its increasingly diverse audience. It has been widely adopted in medical education as a standard evaluation framework – sometimes with modifications and adaptations. The Best Evidence Medical Education Collaborative recommend the use of the Kirkpatrick model in the production of their systematic reviews on medical education.[11,12] The primary benefit of Kirkpatrick's framework is that it pushes the medical education researcher past overly simplistic evaluation methods such as session evaluations and short-term knowledge gain towards longer term outcomes of training in medicine – a change in behaviour (can the learners perform differently as a result of the instruction?) or a change in the ultimate results (even an improvement in patient outcomes). For a medical educator, the process of tying well-written teaching objectives to specific levels in Kirkpatrick's hierarchy can have the benefit of tightly aligning the objectives, instructional strategies, instructional context and assessment methods.

A model that can be used to more broadly examine the curriculum development process is the Context-Inputs-Process-Product (CIPP) model developed by Stufflebeam (Table 26.4).[13] This model was intended by its authors to be used primarily in a formative manner – to improve the implementation of educational projects in process. In this manner, it is useful to assist in the dissemination of novel curricula to other educators as it can highlight development needs, challenges and resources more systematically than an evaluation focussed on learner-focussed results. However, it has also been successfully used summatively to evaluate projects at their conclusion. Its use has been demonstrated in a variety of different health education settings, using a range of data collection methods (from survey and interview to extant data and portfolio review) and targeting learners, faculty and administrators.[13–15] Example research questions formed from the use of the models are presented in Table 26.5.

TABLE 26.4 The CIPP model of educational programme evaluation[13]

Step	Important Questions
Context	What should be done in the project? What are the important contexts and goals for the education?
Inputs	How should the project be done? What are the important resources, personnel and materials required?
Process	How is the project being done? How are the processes working to develop the curriculum? Is the delivery of the education consistent with the plans?
Product	Did the project succeed? Was the curriculum fully developed? Was it implemented successfully? Did the learners achieve the learning objectives?

TABLE 26.5 Example research questions from use of the models

ADDIE	Kirkpatrick	CIPP	Example Research Questions
Analysis	Results	Context	What is the gap between current and desired performance on this topic? For a new educational topic, can goals and objectives be agreed upon across a range of stakeholders?
Design	Knowledge, behaviour	Inputs	What is the baseline level of competency of learners with this topic?
Development		Inputs	What teaching strategies work best for this topic? Which instructional delivery methods work best for this topic: face-to-face, online, self-directed, etc.?
Implementation	Reaction	Process	What resources were required for implementation? What was the experience of the learners?
Evaluation	All steps	Product	Did the learners achieve the educational objectives? Did the learners acquire and sustain new knowledge about the topic? What were the results of this educational project on patient outcomes or provider processes (adjusted for secular trends or compared with a control group)?

RESEARCH METHODS

The diversity of perspective and the comprehensiveness of the evaluation suggested by the types of models described above lend themselves to a broad range of research methods. Quantitative evaluation of outcomes – at the products phase of the CIPP model, or the knowledge, behaviour and results levels of the Kirkpatrick model – are straightforward to consider, but often the hardest to achieve due to constraints on resources, the inability to devise control groups and the confounding of the association between learning and outcome by secular trends and interventions from outside the evaluation. Choice of study design is an important first step setting up a quantitative evaluation, and rigorous evaluation of these outcomes can be performed even in the absence of control groups and randomisation if designed well.[16]

There is a wealth of information to be gained using these models and either mixed or qualitative methods.[17] From the Kirkpatrick model, learner reaction outcomes (Level 1), as well as the attitude, confidence and commitment outcomes at the knowledge level (Level 2), can be obtained by survey, interview and focus group methods. From the CIPP and ADDIE models, curricular goals can be determined by Delphi or focus group methods, faculty development needs can be ascertained by survey or interview and specific questions about of design and development (ADDIE) or inputs and process (CIPP) can be evaluated using survey, interview and focus group.

EXAMPLE

To illustrate the integration of the preceding information, an example – based on a combination of this author's prior experiences in performing and reviewing educational research – may be useful.

Developing social determinants of a health curriculum in a residency programme

Jane and Scott are charged by their programme director with integrating the teaching of social determinants of health (SDoH) into the Family Medicine Residency curriculum. Using the ADDIE framework, they begin with a needs analysis – examining the background literature for information on prevalence, detection and interventions for SDoH in primary care. They consult national curricular standards to define the gap between the residency's current educational practice and the standard. They decide to deploy a validated survey across their regional health system to see which SDoH are most prevalent in their practices. On finding that food insecurity (FI) is the most prevalent SDoH, Scott begins the design and development of a short series of interactive lectures and case-based discussions that will serve as the curriculum and designs a faculty development workshop to prepare for the sessions. He writes specific educational objectives covering screening, referral and patient counselling about FI. Scott plans to gather some immediate reaction data after the didactic sessions to use as formative feedback for his design and develops a short pre- and post-intervention knowledge assessment for the residents (Kirkpatrick Levels 1 and 2, and CIPP – inputs and process).

Jane and Scott discuss the most practical outcome to study for their project and land on the behaviours of screening for FI, and referrals to the residency's social worker and affiliated community health workers (Kirkpatrick Level 3, from Scott's educational objectives). Jane investigates ways to track the frequency of FI screening and referrals using the electronic health record (EHR) and adds a short patient satisfaction survey that she will mail to the clients of the social worker and community health workers. She decides to measure monthly referral rates before and after the educational sessions, and an interrupted time series design to determine if there is a significant lasting impact of the educational sessions on screening and referral practice in the residency. Jane and Scott supplement these measures (using the CIPP framework) with focus group interviews of the faculty and residents, to determine the strengths and weaknesses of the didactic curriculum and the barriers to screening and referral for FI (Process). They also plan a focus group with the social worker and community health workers to determine the impact of the program on their work and gather ideas for further improvement and evaluation of the program (Product).

Along the way, Jane and Scott, having used the curriculum development and evaluation models described above, can produce several potential scholarly reports from their work. Their health system survey on SDoH is potentially of interest to a general medical journal. A report on the full spectrum of Kirkpatrick-level outcomes from the curriculum is of interest to a medical education journal, as is a separate report on the qualitative feedback concerning the curriculum and screening/referral implementation. Finally, a comprehensive review of the curriculum development process, including information about resources, faculty development needs and instructional methods, organised by the ADDIE and/or CIPP frameworks, is suitable for a medical education journal or a presentation at a teaching conference.

CONCLUSION

For each of the models presented in this chapter, there is much written on their individual advantages and limitations. The purpose of the chapter is not to advocate for any specific model, but instead to advocate for the grounding of educational research in established models for curriculum development and evaluation. The use of these types of theoretical frameworks is encouraged for all researchers – in essence, each study result adds to the body of evidence that ultimately validates or refutes the theory.

In the case of educational research, these frameworks lay out the minimum components for an educational project to produce learning and sensible methods to evaluate learner achievement and to understand the success of the project. Educational researchers who do not avail themselves of frameworks like these or others may have unclear goals for their education, and so may have difficulty evaluating their project in a suitable manner. Because of this limitation, their research will often stop at reaction level outcomes, or possibly at short-term knowledge outcomes. Worse yet, they may attempt to evaluate results (Kirkpatrick 4) outcomes without a clear picture of whether the requisite learning and process change is happening (Kirkpatrick Levels 2 and 3) that could produce the change in those outcomes.

Good quality educational research may require multi-step processes for development and evaluation, with multiple potentially researchable questions at each step. Using thoughtful instructional design and evaluation models as a basis for educational development and research will make the work more explicit, and easier to implement and disseminate.

REFERENCES

1. Gustafson KL, Branch RM. *Survey of Instructional Development Models [Internet]*. 4th ed. Syracuse, NY: ERIC Clearinghouse on Information & Technology; 2002 [cited 2020 Jul 29]: 71 p. Available from: https://eric.ed.gov/?q=gustafson+branch&ff1 =subModels&id=ED477517
2. Allen WC. Overview and evolution of the ADDIE training system. *Adv Dev Hum Resour San Franc* 2006 Nov;8(4):430–441.
3. Office of Educational Quality Improvement. *Writing Learning Objectives [Internet]*. Harvard Medical School; 2018 [cited 2020 Aug 5]. Available from: https://meded.hms.harvard.edu/files/hms-med-ed/files/writing_learning_objectives.pdf
4. Butler M, Epstein RA, Totten A, et al. AHRQ series on complex intervention systematic reviews—paper 3: adapting frameworks to develop protocols. *J Clin Epidemiol* 2017 Oct 1;90:19–27.
5. Prideaux D. Curriculum development in medical education: from acronyms to dynamism. *Teach Teach Educ* 2007 Apr 1;23(3):294–302.
6. Harden RM. Learning outcomes and instructional objectives: is there a difference? *Med Teach* 2002 Jan;24(2):151–155.
7. Goldie DJ. AMEE Education Guide no. 29: evaluating educational programmes. *Med Teach* 2006 Jan 1;28(3):210–224.
8. Frye AW, Hemmer PA. Program evaluation models and related theories: AMEE Guide No. 67. *Med Teach* 2012 May 1;34(5):e288–299.
9. Kirkpatrick DL. *Evaluating Training Programs: The Four Levels*. 2nd ed. San Francisco, CA: Berrett-Koehler Publishers; 1998: 289 p.
10. Kirkpatrick JD, Kirkpatrick WK. *Kirkpatrick's Four Levels of Training Evaluation*. Alexandria, VA: ATD Press; 2016: 238 p.
11. Hammick M, Dornan T, Steinert Y. Conducting a best evidence systematic review. Part 1: from idea to data coding. BEME Guide No. 13. *Med Teach* 2010 Jan 1;32(1):3–15.

12. Belfield C, Thomas H, Bullock A, Eynon R, Wall D. Measuring effectiveness for best evidence medical education: a discussion. *Med Teach* 2001 Jan 1;23(2):164–170.
13. Stufflebeam Daniel L. DL. The CIPP model for evaluation. *Int Handb Educ Eval* 2003;31:31–62.
14. Rooholamini A, Amini M, Bazrafkan L, et al. Program evaluation of an Integrated Basic Science Medical Curriculum in Shiraz Medical School, using CIPP evaluation model. *J Adv Med Educ Prof* 2017 Jul;5(3):148–154.
15. Zhang G, Zeller N, Griffith R, et al. Using the context, input, process, and product evaluation model (CIPP) as a comprehensive framework to guide the planning, implementation, and assessment of service-learning programs. *J High Educ Outreach Engagem* 2011;15:57–84.
16. Cochrane Effective Practice and Organisation of Care (EPOC). What study designs can be considered for inclusion in an EPOC review and what should they be called? EPOC Resources for review authors [Internet]. 2017 [cited 2019 Feb 25]. Available from: http://epoc.cochrane.org/resources/epoc-resources-review-authors
17. Schifferdecker KE, Reed VA. Using mixed methods research in medical education: basic guidelines for researchers. *Med Educ* 2009;43(7):637–644.

CHAPTER 27

Programme evaluation

Douglas Archibald

The purpose of this chapter is to help primary care educators and emerging scholars to conduct quality evaluations to improve educational interventions and programmes. Simply put, to help guide the decisions you make to ensure a rigorous evaluation, whether it be for individual teaching sessions, modules or entire programmes. Hopefully, this will help you to structure reports for your leadership teams or accreditation, use the recommendations to propose a new curriculum or even help support a grant application.

There are three sections which lead educators step-by-step through the evaluation process. Part I focusses on what programme evaluation is and what it is not; who it is for and what considerations need to be made, such as using frameworks and logic models. Part II goes through the development of an evaluation plan; and finally Part III deconstructs a primary care education evaluation plan example.

PART I: WHAT DO YOU NEED TO KNOW?
Terminology

Programme evaluation is essentially the determination of whether a programme is working or not, and if there are any unintended consequences.[1] A programme is what you are trying to evaluate ... a workshop, a retreat, a course, a mentoring programme, a curriculum. There are a number of terms used in programme evaluation, and sometimes they are used interchangeably by different people but they do have subtle differences.[2]

- **Assessment** refers to the measurement of knowledge, skills, attitudes, perceptions and behaviours of individuals, groups or even environments. Assessment data can be quantitative (numbers) or qualitative (words), and can be used for different purposes.

- **Evaluation** refers to evaluating programmes designed to produce changes in knowledge, skills, behaviours and other outcomes. The result often leading to recommendations. Evaluation can be *formative* (occurring at various points through programme start-up and delivery; focussing on feedback on the progress and effectiveness of the activities) or *summative* (occurring at a predetermined endpoint and used to assess the overall outcomes of the programme).[3]
- **Research** shares many attributes of evaluation but the goal is different – to create new knowledge which goes beyond local recommendations.

We also need to understand whom the programme evaluation is for. Who are the stakeholders or the audiences? Stakeholders can be funders of the programme, perhaps leadership in your department or staff. They can even be participants in your programme: students, faculty, patients and families.

Evaluation approaches and frameworks

An evaluation framework provides an orientation or blueprint for what needs to be evaluated. It serves as the background for an evaluation plan. Fortunately, there are numerous approaches and frameworks used in health professions education. Before adopting an evaluation approach, you want to consider the intent of the evaluation, stakeholders involved and resources available.[3] While a programme description provides the facts, a programme theory explains how and why a programme is expected to succeed.

We discuss a few of the more common theoretical approaches and frameworks/models used in primary care education: utilisation-focussed approach,[4] participatory/collaborative approaches,[5,6] the CIPP model[7] and Kirkpatrick's hierarchy.[8]

Utilisation-focussed approach
The utilisation-focussed approach focusses the evaluation on the intended use by users of the results or recommendations – usually the decision-makers. The evaluator works with the intended users to determine what kind of evaluation they need. The most appropriate type of evaluation and methods used is based on the needs of the users.

Participatory/collaborative approaches
On the other hand, participatory/collaborative approaches involve all those who have a stake in the programme, including targeted users (students, residents, faculty, perhaps patients), not just funders, policymakers. All stakeholders can be involved in the designing the evaluation questions, collecting and

evaluating data. An example of participatory evaluation is shared later in this chapter. The advantage of this approach is that the recommendations of the evaluation have a high likelihood of being implemented, and all participants will feel a sense of empowerment that builds evaluation capacity within the organisation.[1]

The CIPP model[7,9]

Stufflebeam's Context, Inputs, Processes, Products (CIPP) model is a tool commonly used to evaluate education programmes, large and small. Table 27.1 is an example model taken from the *Incorporating IPCP Teamwork Assessment into Program Evaluation – Practical Guide: Volume 5* (this guide is highly recommended and available to purchase at https://nexusipe.org/advancing/assessment-evaluation/practical-guide).[2]

Using the CIPP model does not prove if a programme works or not, but aims to improve it. Using Table 27.1, we can say that the programme *context* factors listed influence effective teamwork; the *inputs* are appropriate and the *processes* are being implemented; then we should see if the *products* are successful. If this is not the case, then we need to work backwards and ask ourselves questions such as: *Were our products too ambitious? Were our processes not entirely implemented as planned? Were we under resourced (input)?* or *Did we underestimate what needed to be done (inputs)?*

This table is based on a model described in Stufflebeam.[10]

Kirkpatrick's hierarchy[8]

The year 2009 marked 50 years of the four-level Kirkpatrick Model.[11] It involves four levels of evaluation on which to focus questions about the effectiveness of training (Figure 27.1). Over the years, this model has been criticised because evaluators tend to focus on the first two levels which are relatively easy to measure. The model was revised in 2009 to reverse the order of planning a programme to focus on what is most important – programme outcomes. Once the programme has been implemented, the evaluation can occur in their numerical order but not necessarily in a sequential fashion.

Logic models

Logic models are blueprints that graphically represent all the components, activities and anticipated outcomes of a programme. They are tools for conducting theory-driven evaluation[1] (as opposed to specially using a theoretical evaluation approach or model as described previously). Logic models identify the problem or need for the evaluation; the inputs or resources needed for the programme; activities of the programme; outputs (what the programme does with the inputs); outcomes

TABLE 27.1 Example of a CIPP model for an interprofessional team-based simulation programme

Context (What needs to be done?)	Inputs (How should it be done?)	Processes (Is it being done?)	Products (Is it successful?)
• Background, history of simulation programme	• Training philosophy, goals, objectives	• Extent to which programme was fully implemented	Immediate: • Participant satisfaction • Trainer feedback • Change in individual and group proficiency scores
• Teamwork culture at the site level	• Structure of training (length, duration, number of scenarios)	• Participation rates, attrition	Short term: • Group proficiency scores at three months post-training
• Current teamwork processes and evidence of effectiveness	• Simulation resources	• Fidelity of implementation vs. necessary changes	Long term: • Changes in patient satisfaction over one year
• Programme developers' assumption about what needs to change in order for teamwork to improve efficiency and effectiveness	• Staff training • Case scenarios and other materials • Raters and their training • Measurement tools • Requirements, incentives and barriers to participation	• Quality of interactions between trainees, staff and standardised patients	

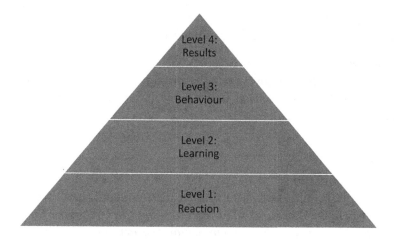

FIGURE 27.1 Four-level Kirkpatrick Model.

(short-term, intermediate and long-term benefits to the learners) and finally impact (system change, and even societal benefit such as improved health care outcomes). See Van Melle https://journals.lww.com/academicmedicine/fulltext/2016/10000/using_a_logic_model_to_assist_in_the_planning,.31.aspx for an excellent open access description of logic models.[12] Conference presentation notes by the same author are also publically available on the Royal College of Physicians and Surgeons Canada website at http://www.royalcollege.ca/rcsite/documents/icre/competency-based-education-vanmelle.pdf and may be of benefit.[13]

PART II: HOW DO YOU DO IT?

Before conducting an evaluation, it is a good idea to have an evaluation plan. Much of this section comes from the *Incorporating IPCP Teamwork Assessment into Program Evaluation – Practical Guide: Volume 5*.[2] You need to consider (a) the context, (b) design decisions and (c) implementation logistics.

Context

Programme rationale

This is simply your elevator pitch. Why is your programme/innovation needed? What issues/challenges/problems are you trying to address?

Programme description

Include details such as programme name, length or duration, goals, objectives, materials and assessments.

Programme theory

What assumptions guide the programme (see Part I)?

Evaluation purpose

What do you need to know about the programme that you do not know already? What decisions need to be made based on the findings of the evaluation?

Design decisions

Evaluation questions

What are you trying to find out? Example questions could be: *Is your training programme different at rural and urban training sites? What are the barriers and facilitators to implementing your mentoring programme?* and *What aspects of this faculty development programme had a positive impact on teaching at your institution?*

Required information

What information will best answer you evaluation questions?

Information source

Who is the best source for the required information?

Study methods

Who will collect the information and how? It is important to note that evaluation and research share many of the designs and methods. If you are new to evaluation and do not have research experience, you may want to consult with an expert in your locale. For example, if you are collecting data from different groups but over the same time period, you may want to use a *cross-sectional design*. If you are collecting data from the same group over time, you may want to consider a *cohort design*. There are many measurement tools in the methods toolbox for you to choose: knowledge tests, surveys, interviews, focus groups, Simulated Office Oral Exams (SOOs), performance evaluations, chart reviews and the list goes on.

Analytic procedures

How will the data you collect be analysed? A good evaluator will determine the analysis a priori. Again, talk with a local researcher to help you with the analysis as well as the methods. *Qualitative* data analysis generated from interviews and focus groups, for example, can include thematic content analysis, frequency analysis and coding (both inductive and deductive). *Quantitative* data analysis from surveys, tests and other measurement tools can include descriptive and inferential statistics. Consult a researcher or statistician if available.

Interpretation

Data do not necessarily speak for themselves. Good evaluators will discuss the findings and results with their stakeholders. Many times interpreting data can be subjective but it is possible to implement benchmarks or standards ahead of time. Perhaps success may be for participants to achieve 80% of a given criteria, or for the programme to reduce training costs by 10%.

Implementation logistics

Management of the evaluation

You should identify who on your evaluation team will do what. Think of the components of an evaluation: design, ethical study conduct, budget, management, creation and implementation of the evaluation plan and dissemination of the findings.

Timelines

Just as important as *who* will do what is *when*. Drawing up a timeline is very important. Be sure all stakeholders have input into the timeline.

Reporting

To whom and how should you share the findings and recommendations of the report? Consult the Communication and Reporting chapter of *Program Evaluation Standards: A Guide for Evaluators and Evaluation Users*, pp. 217–224.[14] There are lots of great tips like scheduling informal and formal reporting during the evaluation determined by information users' needs, and selecting or creating guidelines to ensure formal reports are accurate.

PART III: WHAT DOES IT LOOK LIKE? EXAMPLES FROM PRIMARY CARE

An example evaluation is a Pan-Canadian one that I co-lead. The Executive Summary of the final report reproduced below includes all elements of the evaluation plan. The programme evaluated can be found here: https://www.cfpc.ca/uploadedFiles/Education/_PDFs/FTA_GUIDE_TM_ENG_Apr15_REV.pdf

FTA framework analysis of awareness and application: final report

The purpose of this study was to evaluate the awareness, uptake and utilisation of the Fundamental Teaching Activities Framework (here within referred to as the FTA framework) in Canadian departments of family medicine, their educational programmes and by family medicine teachers. This report is provide the College of Family Medicine Canada (CFPC), in particular the Faculty Development Education Committee (FDEC) with an understanding of the degree of awareness, application, integration and potential impact of the FTA framework on faculty development directors (FDDs), postgraduate programme directors (PDs) and site directors (SDs).

Using a two-part mixed methods design, we first formed an expert panel consisting of the research team plus three members of FDEC. The first part of the design required us to create a survey to be sent to all 17 family medicine institutions across the country. The survey was crafted by the research team and then reviewed and edited by the entire expert panel. Final surveys were created in both English and French.

In Part I, the survey was converted into an electronic form and distributed to the institutions on 7 September 2018 to be completed by each institution's FDD, PD and SDs. The survey closed on 23 November 2018. In total 12/15 FDDs, 12/18 PDs and 34/174 SDs responded to the surveys; resulting in 80%, 66.7% and 19.5% response rates, respectively. This constitutes an overall response rate of 28%.

In Part II, all FDDs, PDs and SDs were invited to participate in a semi-structured interview to elaborate on the survey results (conducted over the telephone or ZOOM, lasting up to 60 minutes). The interview protocols are included in the appendix of this report. Interviews were conducted over a five-month period from January to May 2019. In total, 15 interviews (6 FDDs, 3 PDs and 3 SDs) were conducted and transcripts analysed.

The findings of the interviews were categorised as individual values; collective values; the organization and clarity of the FTA framework; use of the framework; suggested interventions to improve its use and limitations.

Key findings from the surveys and interviews

- The FTA framework is conceptually sound, with the content laid out with good clarity and in a well-organised manner.
- The main facilitators for its utilisation include, but are not limited to, faculty development and promote teaching activities in family medicine.
- Areas of improvement to the document, in an attempt to convey the framework's content in a user-friendly fashion for preceptors.
- A number of suggested interventions were highlighted, in hopes of promoting the implementation of FTA concepts towards resident training or preceptor evaluation in clinical teaching.

REFERENCES

1. Lovato C, Peterson L. Programme evaluation. In: Swanwick T, Forrest K, O'Brien B, eds. *Understanding Medical Education: Evidence, Theory, and Practice*. 3rd ed. John Wiley & Sons, Ltd.; Milton, Australia. 2019: 443–455.
2. Schmitz C, Collins L, Michalec B, Archibald D. *Incorporating IPCP Teamwork Assessment into Program Evaluation Practical Guide*. Vol. 5. Minnesota, USA: Center for Interpofessional Practice and Education; 2017.

3. Archibald D, MacDonald C, Bajnok I, Puddester D. Practice outcomes and measuring success with interprofessional practice. In: Coffey S, Anyinam C, eds. *Interprofessional Healthcare Practice*. Canada: Pearson; 2014: 208–230.

4. Patton M, Patton M. *Essentials of Utilization-Focused Evaluation*. 1st ed. Sage Publications: Thousand Oaks, CA, USA. 2011.

5. Cousins JB. *Collaborative Approaches to Evaluation*. Sage Publications; London, UK. 2019.

6. Cousins JB, Earl L. The case for participatory evaluation: theory, research, practice. In: Cousins J, Earl L, eds. *Participatory Evaluation in Education: Studies in Evaluation Use and Organizational Learning*. Falmer; London, UK. 1995: 3–18. Available from: http://legacy.oise.utoronto.ca/research/field-centres/ross/ctl1014/Cousins1995.pdf (Accessed 29 June 2020).

7. Stufflebeam D. The CIPP model for program evaluation. In: Madaus GF, Scriven MS, Stufflebeam DL, eds. *Evaluation Models: Viewpoints on Educational and Human Services Evaluation. Evaluation in Education and Human Services*. Netherlands: Springer; 1983:117–141. doi:10.1007/978-94-009-6669-7_7

8. Kirkpatrick D. Evaluation of training. In: Craig RL, Bittel LR, eds. *Training and Development Handbook*. McGraw-Hill: New York, USA. 1967: 87–112.

9. Kellaghan T, Stufflebeam DL, eds. *International Handbook of Educational Evaluation: Part One: Perspectives/Part Two: Practice*. Netherlands: Springer; 2003. doi:10.1007/978-94-010-0309-4

10. Stufflebeam D. The CIPP model for evaluation. In: Stufflebeam DL, Madaus GF, Kellaghan T, eds. *Evaluation Models*. Springer; The Netherlands. 2000: 279–317.

11. Kirkpatrick JD, Kirkpatrick WK. *Kirkpatrick's Four Levels of Training Evaluation*. USA: Association for Talent Development Press; 2016.

12. Van Melle E. Using a logic model to assist in the planning, implementation, and evaluation of educational programs. *Acad Med* 2016;91(10):1464. doi:10.1097/ACM.0000000000001282

13. Van Melle E, Flynn L, Kaba A, Tavares W, Horsley T. Program Evaluation for Competency-based medical Education: Are we making a difference? Presented at the: 2016 International Conference on Residency Education; 29 September 2016.

14. Yarbrough DB. Joint Committee on Standards for Educational Evaluation. In: *The Program Evaluation Standards: A Guide for Evaluators and Evaluation Users*. 3rd ed. Sage: Thousand Oaks, CA, USA. 2011.

CHAPTER 28

Researching the informal and hidden curriculum

Hilary Neve

WHAT DO WE MEAN BY THE HIDDEN CURRICULUM?

The hidden curriculum is an umbrella term describing the learning, often unintended, which takes place outside of the formal, planned, taught curriculum. Hafferty identified two main elements[1] (Box 28.1). A recent scoping review highlights the ambiguous and interchangeable use of terms such as 'informal' and 'hidden' within the literature, and emphasises the importance of researchers clarifying which aspect of the hidden curriculum they are studying, as well as the specific context in which they are doing so.[2]

Given its impact on learners, ongoing research is vital, to ensure that we reduce the negative effects and harness the positive elements of the hidden curriculum. Many teachers and clinicians remain unaware of its existence and impact, and the hidden curriculum is not widely studied in primary care.[3]

WHY DOES THE HIDDEN CURRICULUM MATTER?

The hidden curriculum can have a powerful impact on the development of learners, shaping their professional identity and socialising them into what is 'actually' valued and what is acceptable or unacceptable in medical education and health care practice.[8,10] Negative experiences may lead to a reduction in empathy,[11] idealism,[12] ethical erosion[13] as well as influencing career choice. Tensions between the taught and informal curriculum can lead students to feel powerless, pessimistic and conflicted,[6] particularly where unprofessional behaviours are tolerated.[12] Importantly, the hidden curriculum can also be a

BOX 28.1   DEFINING THE HIDDEN CURRICULUM

The hidden curriculum is context-specific and often seen as having two elements[1] which may interact:

Informal curriculum: the ad hoc, unscripted and usually unarticulated learning[4] that occurs independently of the formal curriculum, for example, through day-to-day interactions with, and observation of, role models:

- *Repeatedly hearing the term 'just a GP' may lead learners to see general practitioners as of lower status than hospital doctors.*[5]
- *Observing health professionals making time to understand a patient's perspective can enhance learners' patient-centred attitudes.*[6]

Hidden curriculum: the set of influences communicated to learners (1) by the structure and culture of academic and health organisations (e.g. medical schools, general practices and hospitals) and (2) by the curriculum content, what is included, prioritised and what is assessed. This includes the messages communicated by the 'null' curriculum – subjects which are left out.[7]

- *If assessments focus primarily on biomedical learning, learners may come to see humanistic and professional elements of medicine as of secondary importance.*[8] *If trainees see consultants, but not GPs, being promoted to senior academic roles, this may perpetuate the belief that general practice is less intellectually stimulating.*[9]

positive influence,[14] complementing and enhancing learning from the formal curriculum. This is an under-researched area[2] which could usefully be studied within primary care.

HOW CAN STUDYING THE HIDDEN CURRICULUM IN PRIMARY CARE BE USEFUL?

Most research to date has taken place in medical undergraduate settings. Evidence suggests, however, that hidden curriculum issues extend across all stages of training and across professions.[12] Given the lack of research within primary care, initial qualitative exploratory studies, using methods such as a cultural web,[15] could identify key elements of the hidden curriculum for trainees and clinicians. The informal curriculum is particularly important in primary care where much learning, for example, around communication, teamworking, professionalism, cultural competence[3] and patient-centredness, occurs through observing and listening to health professionals at work, rather than through formal teaching. Exploring the factors that help and hinder such learning could be an exciting area for future research.

At an undergraduate level, researchers have used a range of qualitative[16,17] and quantitative[18,19] approaches to explore the factors, including implicit messages from role models and peers, that shape medical students' perceptions of general practice. Future research could explore specific negative messages in more depth, or study ways of harnessing the hidden curriculum to counteract these messages. For example, students often state that general practice is not intellectually stimulating. What do students actually mean by this? And how could general practitioners employ the informal curriculum to better articulate and demonstrate the academic challenges?

Research could also explore the impact of the hidden curriculum on those concepts which may be fundamental or 'special' to thinking and practising effectively in primary care.[20,21] These are concepts around which trainees and students often have negative perceptions, such as managing uncertainty, patients with chronic pain[22] and complexity, or addressing population as well as individual needs. In what ways does the informal curriculum help or hinder learners' ability to accept and manage these issues in primary care? Do even subtle differences in language (e.g. using terms such as 'managing' or 'embracing' rather than 'tolerating' when defining learning outcomes around uncertainty) influence students' perceptions?

WHAT APPROACHES AND METHODOLOGIES COULD BE USEFUL?

Hidden curriculum literature from different contexts, particularly undergraduate medicine, can illustrate useful approaches and methodologies.

1. *Understanding learners' experiences of the informal and hidden curriculum*

    Most researchers use qualitative studies, such as semi-structured interviews,[23,24] focus groups[6] or analysis of students' written reflections.[25] These can provide rich and authentic insights, particularly where learners are asked to recall and reflect on specific hidden curriculum experiences. However, they have limited generalisability. 'Straight after the moment' audio-diaries can be easy for learners to use and avoid the risk of hindsight bias.[26] The tacit nature of the hidden curriculum can be problematic, as learners may not notice the influences upon them. Some researchers introduce students to the notion of the hidden curriculum first,[14,25] or ask learners to describe events where they felt emotional or conflicted. Others ask about specific areas, such as learners' experiences of discriminatory behaviour[27] or nutrition learning.[23]

Initial exploratory questionnaires, as well as literature reviews, can help inform interview questions.[24]

Quantitative methods can provide information about frequency and subgroup differences.[18] Observational studies (e.g. observing clinical teaching sessions) can identify positive and negative examples of the informal curriculum which learners and teachers may have not noticed, as well as missed teaching opportunities.[28]

2. *Exploring the impact of the informal and hidden curriculum on learners*

Most researchers rely on learner perceptions, using qualitative methods to explore how they believe experiences have influenced their identity formation,[29] how they felt when informal learning experiences conflicted with formal teaching[6] or how they decided to adopt or reject messages or adapted their behaviour.[24,25] A limitation is that learners may not recognise how hidden influences have affected them; comparison with trainers' perceptions can strengthen the findings. Quantitative tools can be used to measure changes in learner empathy, or how their perceptions of unprofessional behaviour change as they progress through a course.[30]

3. *Researching the effectiveness of initiatives to address the negative or harness the positive effects of the hidden curriculum*

Attempts to minimise the negative impact of the hidden curriculum often involve training faculty and shifting organisational culture, but this is under-researched. Initiatives to reveal the hidden curriculum to learners, encouraging them to notice and reflect on these experiences,[14,25] could be implemented and studied within primary care. The impact of increasing trainers' awareness of this issue and whether, and how, they then become change agents in tackling the hidden curriculum is another possible area of study.[6]

PARTICULAR ISSUES TO CONSIDER WHEN RESEARCHING THE HIDDEN AND INFORMAL CURRICULUM

Clear guidance around confidentiality and anonymity is vital to ensure learners feel able to share sensitive information, such as experiences of unprofessional practice. Using trained student or trainee interviewers may increase participants' sense of safety,[11] or the social support of focus groups may help overcome any reluctance to share examples of poor practice.[29]

Triangulation can improve the reliability of research findings, for example, following up observatory studies with interviews where participants reflect on the observed events, or interviewing both trainers and trainees and comparing and contrasting their responses.

Clinicians may themselves be socialised into aspects of the hidden curriculum; as a result they may take issues raised by research data for granted or not identify them as important. Having a collaborative approach to analysis with external perspectives on the team can help avoid this. Including patients and students or trainees in the research team can also bring important perspectives.

CONCLUSION

Researching the hidden and informal curriculum is not without its challenges, but it may provide valuable insights for primary care education. Sharing research findings with trainers, or using findings to inform policy or curriculum change, could help enhance the quality of student and trainee education and improve patient care. Such changes might also improve learners' perceptions of general practice; longer term this might help address workload problems in primary care.

REFERENCES

1. Hafferty F. Beyond curriculum reform: confronting medicine's hidden curriculum. *Acad Med* 1998;73(4):403–407.
2. Lawrence C, Mhlaba T, Stewart KA, Moletsane R, Gaede B, Moshabela M. The hidden curricula of medical education: a scoping review. *Acad Med* 2018 Apr;93(4):648–656.
3. Rothlind E, Fors U, Salminen H, Wändell P, Ekblad S. The informal curriculum of family medicine–what does it entail and how is it taught to residents? A systematic review. *BMC Fam Pract* 2020 Dec;21:149 doi.org/10.1186/s12875-020-01120-1
4. Cribb A, Bignold S. Towards a reflexive medical school: the hidden curriculum and medical education research. *Stud Higher Educ* 1999;24(2):195–208.
5. Wass V, Gregory S. Not 'just' a GP: a call for action. *Br J Gen Pract* 2017;67(657):148–149.
6. White CB, Kumagai AK, Ross PT, Fantone JC. A qualitative exploration of how the conflict between the formal and informal curriculum influences student values and behaviors. *Acad Med* 2009 May 1;84(5):597–603.
7. Flinders DJ, Noddings N, Thornton SJ. The null curriculum: its theoretical basis and practical implications. *Curric Inq* 1986 Mar 1;16(1):33–42.
8. Martimianakis MA, Michalec B, Lam J, Cartmill C, Taylor JS, Hafferty FW. Humanism, the hidden curriculum, and educational reform: a scoping review and thematic analysis. *Acad Med* 2015 Nov 1;90(11):S5–13.
9. Wass V, Gregory S, Petty-Saphon K. *By Choice—Not By Chance: Supporting Medical Students Towards Future Careers in General Practice.* London: Health Education England and the Medical Schools Council; Mar 2016.
10. Haldet P. The role of the student-teacher relationship in the formation of physicians. *J Gen Intern Med* 2006;21:S16–20.
11. Eikeland HL, Ørnes K, Finset A, Pedersen R. The physician's role and empathy – a qualitative study of third year medical students. *BMC Med Educ* 2014 Dec;14(1):1–8.
12. Doja A, Bould MD, Clarkin C, Eady K, Sutherland S, Writer H. The hidden and informal curriculum across the continuum of training: a cross-sectional qualitative study. *Med Teach* 2016 Apr 2;38(4):410–418.
13. Lehmann LS, Sulmasy LS, Desai S. Hidden curricula, ethics, and professionalism: optimizing clinical learning environments in becoming and being a physician: a position paper of the American College of Physicians. *Ann Int Med* 2018 Apr 3;168(7):506–508.
14. Neve H, Collett T. Empowering students with the hidden curriculum. *Clin Teach* 2018 Dec;15(6):494–499.

15. Mossop L, Dennick R, Hammond R, Robbé I. Analysing the hidden curriculum: use of a cultural web. *Med Educ* 2013 Feb;47(2):134–143.

16. Reid K, Alberti H. Medical students' perceptions of general practice as a career; a phenomenological study using socialisation theory. *Educ Prim Care* 2018;29(4):208–214.

17. Nicholson S, Hastings AM, McKinley RK. Influences on students' career decisions concerning general practice: a focus group study. *Br J Gen Pract* 2016 Oct 1;66(651):e768–775.

18. Royal College of General Practitioners. Medical Schools Council. Destination GP. Medical students' experiences and perceptions of general practice; 2017. Available from: https://www.rcgp.org.uk/-/media/Files/Policy/A-Z-policy/2017/RCGP-destination-GP-nov-2017.ashx?la=en

19. Gami M, Howe A. Experience adds up! Questionnaire study: attitudes of medical students towards a career in general practice. *Educ Prim Care* 2020 Mar 3;31(2):89–97.

20. Neve H. Learning to become a primary care professional: insights from threshold concept theory. *Educ Prim Care* 2019 Jan 2;30(1):5–8.

21. Vaughan K. Vocational thresholds: developing expertise without certainty in general practice medicine. *J Prim Health Care* 2016 Jun 1;8(2):99–105.

22. Corrigan C, Desnick L, Marshall S, Bentov N, Rosenblatt RA. What can we learn from first-year medical students' perceptions of pain in the primary care setting? *Pain Med* 2011 Aug 1;12(8):1216–1222.

23. Martin S, Sturgiss E, Douglas K, Ball L. Hidden curriculum within nutrition education in medical schools. *BMJ Nutr Prevent Health* 2020. bmjnph-2019-000059. doi:10.1136/bmjnph-2019-000059

24. Hill E, Bowman K, Stalmeijer R, Hart J. You've got to know the rules to play the game: how medical students negotiate the hidden curriculum of surgical careers. *Med Educ.* 2014 Sep;48(9):884–894.

25. Gaufberg EH, Batalden M, Sands R, Bell SK. The hidden curriculum: what can we learn from third-year medical student narrative reflections? *Acad Med* 2010 Nov 1;85(11):1709–1716.

26. Neve H, Lloyd H, Collett T. Understanding students' experiences of professionalism learning: a 'threshold' approach. *Teach Higher Educ* 2017 Jan 2;22(1):92–108.

27. Phillips SP, Clarke M. More than an education: the hidden curriculum, professional attitudes and career choice. *Med Educ* 2012 Sep;46(9):887–893.

28. Gray A, Enright H. Opening the black box: an observational study of teaching and learning interactions for paediatrics trainees on consultant ward rounds. *J Paed Child Health* 2018 Sep;54(9):1011–1015.

29. Silveira GL, Campos LK, Schweller M, Turato ER, Helmich E, de Carvalho-Filho MA. "Speed up"! The influences of the hidden curriculum on the professional identity development of medical students. *Health Prof Educ* 2019 Sep 1;5(3):198–209.

30. Reddy ST, Farnan JM, Yoon JD, et al. Third-year medical students' participation in and perceptions of unprofessional behaviors. *Acad Med* 2007 Oct 1;82(10):S35–39.

CHAPTER 29

Mentoring: how to support and mentor early researchers in educational research

David Ponka

In most contexts, where funding for clinical care and biomedical research is often a significant percentage of health care spending, support for medical education research is often lacking.[1] The problem is compounded in low-middle-income countries where scarcer resources go to fill pressing needs, as opposed to evaluation and innovation of medical education which is an investment for the future.

Even in high-income countries, institutions seeking to build capacity in research in general, let alone medical education research, are few. One study estimated institutions in the United States taking on such a 'replicative' role at only 3%.[2]

Research training as part of clinical training is a relatively new concept. Some key guidelines are useful to help a medical education mentor, trying to assist a new scholar in the discipline. See Box 29.1 for an exemplar in Guyana.

WHAT WORKS AND WHAT TO AVOID?

When mentoring learners and faculty new to research in a medical education scholarship project, three phrases may prove useful.

1. *'Focus, focus, focus': it all begins with the research question*
   Too often, new researchers propose questions that are important, but may not be focussed enough to be achievable or to provide specific

BOX 29.1 EXEMPLAR: GUYANA

Family medicine is a new specialty in Guyana, but every effort has been made to enshrine research as part of the nascent discipline. Developing research capacity has taken concerted effort, above all because of the seemingly limitless clinical demands. However, these efforts were made because of the foresight that research and specifically medical education research could also confer efficiencies at the academic practice level, as well as pay dividends as residents entered practice throughout the country.

The programme has formed a relationship with Academics Without Borders (AWB) aimed to start train-the-trainer research skills workshops for faculty. AWB adopts a microresearch paradigm that permits clinician teachers to work at the practice level and answer a research question that has immediate impact and that can be incorporated into everyday needs.

guidance on the area of interest. *What is the situation with regards to research training during residency education in my country?* is too broad. *How do current trainees in postgraduate family medicine in my university feel their research training and mentorship could be improved to increase their likelihood to continue in research?* is much better – and achievable for a new researcher.

2. *'What are you passionate about?': research takes times and energy*

    Many medical education researchers are often clinicians and teachers first. The demands of patient care are constant and take priority. Research will often occur in evenings, on weekends, or over holidays. This is why the research question has to be of great interest to the early researcher and promise a tangible result likely to improve their every-day practice or teaching (see Box 29.2).

3. *'Research is a team sport': beyond individual mentorship*

    Most significant research is achieved through sustained partnerships to examine a question in depth. Yet, many universities continue to require that their students work from independent data sets that they have acquired alone. This is not how the real world works. We encourage trainees and new researchers to work in teams to achieve sustained results. Trainees, even if unable to work in dyads, can often work on related questions or build on another trainee's previous work. University research networks are an important way to link emerging researchers to more established ones, and will often ask the most relevant question for a particular training context.

BOX 29.2   MICRORESEARCH[3,4] AND IMPLEMENTATION SCIENCE[5]

Many leading research capacity-building organisations, such as AWB, espouse a microresearch paradigm which focussed on achievable results by asking simple, locally relevant research questions. Another important paradigm is implementation science which challenges us to focus on research that will lead to implementation of a proven interventions (e.g. educational innovation) in a particular context.

REMOTE MENTORSHIP

Truly emerging settings may not have access to local mentors and in this instance, an international collaboration can prove fruitful. This carries some risk as the local perspective and an understanding of needs are key. In this sense, the mentor should be as knowledgeable of the local reality as possible.

The global COVID-19 pandemic and environmental pressures are making traveling less appealing, however, and many institutions are pivoting towards virtual education. Scholarship in this area is thus very timely, as is a better understanding of how to mentor medical education research at a distance. Clearly, a train-the-trainer and capacity-building approach, building in a layer of mentorship at the local level ('mentoring a mentor') becomes even more important.[6]

CONCLUSIONS

Mentoring a learner or colleague in medical education research can be very rewarding and impactful, as it can have exponentially additive effects. As in other types of teaching and mentorship, enthusiasm for the material and project, as well as establishing a relationship based on trust that we have the mentees best interests at heart, are key.

Focussing a medical education research question, and ensuring its applicability to the local context, is critical as well. What is sometimes less obvious is to successfully embed a mentee into an existing research team. This ensures that the mentee develops the team work skills, in addition to the technical skills, that research requires. The established research team will benefit from the addition of a fresh, often current, perspective as well.

Indeed, research divorced from a pragmatic perspective can lack relevance, just as a practice or a teaching team without embedded researchers risks being less informed of evidence.

FURTHER ONLINE RESOURCES:

AAMC Research in Medical Education: https://www.aamc.org/system/files/c/2/429856-mededresearchprimer.pdf

A list of leading Medical Education Journals: https://www.mcgill.ca/medicinefacdev/links/journals

Academics Without Borders: https://www.awb-usf.org/

Microresearch framework: http://www.microresearch.ca/how-it-works

12 tips for both mentors and mentees/students[7]: https://www.mededpublish.org/manuscripts/400

REFERENCES

1. Asch DA, Weinstein DF. Innovation in medical education. *N Engl J Med* 2014;371:794–795.
2. Ewigman B, Davis A, Vansaghi T, et al. Building research & scholarship capacity in departments of family medicine: a new joint ADFM-NAPCRG initiative. *Ann Fam Med* 2016;14(1):82–83. doi:10.1370/afm.1901
3. Microresearch. *How it works.* Available from: http://www.microresearch.ca/how-it-works (Accessed 24 June 2020).
4. MacDonald NE, Bortolussi R, Kabakyenga J, et al. MicroResearch: finding sustainable local health solutions in East Africa through small local research studies. *J Epidemiol Glob Health* 2014;4(3):185–193. doi:10.1016/j.jegh.2014.01.002
5. Price DW, Wagner DP, Krane NK, et al. What are the implications of implementation science for medical education? *Med Educ Online* 2015;20:27003.
6. Ponka D, Coffman M, Fraser K et al. Fostering global primary care research: a capacity-building approach. *BMJ Glob Health.* 2020, 5:e002470
7. Barnard J, Ledger A. Practical tips for undertaking a medical education research project and the undergraduate level: Recommendations for both students and supervisors. *MedEdPublish* 2016;5:27.

CHAPTER 30

How to develop critical mass and ensure primary care educational innovations and initiatives are evidence-based

*Bob Mash and
Jan de Maeseneer*

INTRODUCTION

This chapter looks at how educational research can support the development of family medicine and primary care education in a country or region. We reflect on our experience within the PRIMAFAMED (Primary Care and Family Medicine) network over the last 20 years[1] and how educational research has enabled the development of family medicine and primary care in sub-Saharan Africa. From this experience, we share lessons and ideas that have applicability to other countries and regions.

The PRIMAFAMED network includes 40 academic institutions across the region within low-, low-middle and upper-middle-income countries. The African continent has 25% of the global disease burden, but only 3% of the world's health workers and less than 1% of the world's health expenditure.[2] Within this context, there has been a sustained focus on developing family medicine and primary care education and educational research has been a key part of the process.

In thinking about the development of family medicine and primary care education, we have adopted the 'stages of change' model to make sense of where different countries are in the process.[3] Each stage in this process has different challenges to overcome in order to move forward[4]:

- *Pre-contemplation*: Countries are not considering the introduction of family medicine education and training.

Contemplation: The key role players are actively considering the need for family medicine education and training. Three key role players are the ministry of health, which creates policy for the health system; universities or colleges, which have to conduct training programmes and the council or registration body, which has to accredit and register the new qualifications and graduates. Advocates for family medicine are often located in medical schools, professional bodies or civil society organisations within the country.

- *Preparation*: Once the key role players agree on the need for training programmes, the educational institutions need to design and develop these. This process starts with an analysis of the context, and how the graduates of the training programme will contribute to the local health system. If there are several institutions involved, it is preferable that key aspects of the curriculum are agreed upon nationally. This is not always an easy process, as ethnic, religious, political and historical differences may be difficult to overcome.
- *Action*: The educational institutions launch the training programmes and enrol the first students. It often takes several years before the first graduates are produced and enter the health system, and a reliable pipeline is created.
- *Maintenance*: Once the country has a reliable pipeline of new graduates entering the health system, it is necessary to ensure that appropriate posts are created, that graduates are making a difference and fulfilling the intended roles, adjusting the expected roles if necessary and ensuring alignment between human resources for health policy and training capacity.

EDUCATIONAL RESEARCH AND THE DEVELOPMENT OF TRAINING

Each of the stages described above generates a number of key educational questions which can be addressed through research (Table 30.1). Educational research can be a key catalyst in the process, and should be embraced at each stage of change. In the sections below, we use the example of postgraduate training in family medicine, but the same principles apply to the introduction of family medicine in undergraduate programmes or internship, as well as for other novel primary care education initiatives such as for physician assistants or nurse practitioners.

TABLE 30.1 Education research questions and methods aligned with the stages of change model for postgraduate family medicine training

Stage of Change	Key Educational Questions for Initiation of Postgraduate Family Medicine Training	Typical Research Methods	Examples
Pre-contemplation	How to create a conversation with policymakers on the need for family medicine training?	Knowledge translation of evidence from elsewhere.	A scoping review described the current status of family medicine in sub-Saharan Africa and mapped existing evidence of its strengths, weaknesses, effectiveness and impact.[6]
Contemplation	How to present evidence to policy and decision makers? What can family medicine contribute to the health system? Can we afford specialists in family medicine in the health system?	Knowledge translation of evidence from elsewhere. Delphi studies to obtain consensus on contribution to the health system. Exploratory qualitative studies to understand the perspective of key stakeholders.	Using the Delphi method to reach regional consensus on the key principles of family medicine in Africa.[9] Exploring the views of key stakeholders prior to the launch of family medicine training in Zimbabwe.[7]
Preparation	What are the intended learning outcomes of training? What is the most appropriate design of the training programme? How to develop a supportive learning environment?	Scoping reviews that synthesise relevant evidence to guide planning. Delphi studies to obtain consensus on learning outcomes and clinical skills. Reports on workshops that define concepts and reach consensus on key issues.	A scoping review led to the creation of a model for decentralised training in low- and middle-income countries.[15] Use of the Delphi method to reach consensus on national learning outcomes for all training programmes.[13]

(Continued)

TABLE 30.1 (*Continued*)

Stage of Change	Key Educational Questions for Initiation of Postgraduate Family Medicine Training	Typical Research Methods	Examples
Action	Is the training programme working? How can we improve the training programme?	Case studies or surveys of training programmes. Experimental studies that evaluate the effect of training and innovations.	A survey of first cohort of students in the Gezira Family Medicine Project, Sudan.[17] A quasi-experimental study evaluating the introduction of an e-portfolio for workplace-based learning and assessment.[19]
Maintenance	What happens to our graduates? Are family physicians making a difference in the health system? How to align training outputs with policy on human resources for health in the health system?	Surveys of graduates and family physicians. Observational studies of family physicians in the health system. Phenomenology. Exploratory qualitative studies with key stakeholders. Analysis of human resources for health data.	A survey of recent graduates to determine career path and feedback on training.[22] An observational study comparing facilities with and without family physicians.[24] A qualitative exploration of how district managers viewed the introduction of family physicians.[25]

Pre-contemplation

Countries that are not contemplating postgraduate family medicine have no active educational research questions. Advocates of family medicine, however, need evidence from other countries to initiate a conversation with policymakers. Such evidence needs to address issues such as the impact and cost-effectiveness of specialists in family medicine within similar health systems. Evidence generated in countries that are at the maintenance stage is most useful here, and puts a responsibility on these countries at a later stage of development to provide such evidence. Evidence coming from similar contexts is also important. In sub-Saharan Africa, it is difficult to convince policymakers with evidence from Europe or the United States of America where the resources and models of primary care are very different. Evidence needs to be generated from countries with a similar level of resources and comparable district health systems. For example, an analysis of African leaders' views on critical human resource issues revealed that they favoured a district health system with a key role for family medicine.[5] Local advocates need skills in synthesising and translating this evidence into forms that policymakers can engage with. Scoping reviews can synthesise relevant evidence on how family medicine is being implemented and practiced in the region,[6] and disseminated to policymakers in the form of issue or policy briefs.

Contemplation

The dialogue with key stakeholders continues in this stage, as advocates address ambivalence and uncertainty. The need to synthesise and translate evidence from elsewhere continues. Key educational questions can, however, be usefully addressed in the local context. It may be helpful to explore what key stakeholders are actually thinking and what their concerns are with regard to family medicine.[7,8] Descriptive exploratory qualitative research can be invaluable in this regard and the findings can inform the debate. Such stakeholders include policy- and decision makers as well as other disciplines, patients and community representatives.

It may also be helpful to clarify in the local country context what roles family physicians might play in the health system. For example, should they be placed at district and primary hospitals, or in primary care facilities, or both? To what extent will family physicians be involved in management and administration of health services? Achieving consensus on this between advocates, policymakers, academics, managers and providers can be assisted by educational research. Consensus and prioritisation methods such as the Delphi technique and nominal group technique can be valuable.[9,10]

Preparation

Once the decision to approve training has been made, then educational institutions must design and develop the training programmes. A number of educational research questions arise at this point. For example, what are the intended programmatic learning outcomes, competencies and clinical skills? If there are multiple new programmes in a country, it is also helpful to address these questions collectively and have national outcomes that all programmes align with. Again, methods that build consensus and prioritise are valuable.[11-13] Workshops may be held within the country to think through the design of different components of the curriculum, and these can be reported as they define key conceptual thinking and consensus amongst stakeholders.[14]

Programmes may still differ in their educational approach, and will plan appropriate content, resources, training sites, teachers and trainers. Scoping reviews may assist with gathering evidence on what has worked elsewhere, for example, with developing effective learning environments on the distributed platform.[15] Family medicine training often uses parts of the health system that are not used by other specialist training programmes, more based in teaching hospitals. The distributed platform, which may consist of communities, primary care facilities and district hospitals, may not have experience with such postgraduate specialist training. Research can help to define what is needed to create a supportive interprofessional learning environment.[16]

Action

Once training programmes are initiated and rolled out over several years until the first cohort of students has graduated, there may be a variety of educational research questions. Stakeholders will want to know if the training programmes are working and what needs to be improved. Programmes may be subjected to external accreditation and receive feedback on their performance. However, in the early stages, more formal research may also be useful to gauge how students, teachers and trainers are experiencing the programme, and to identify strengths and weaknesses.[17]

Innovations are often introduced as the training programme is consolidated and need to be evaluated and shared with others. For example, the development of a paper-based portfolio for workplace-based learning and assessment[18] and subsequent conversion to an electronic portfolio.[19] Evaluation of such innovations may involve mixed methods, for example, experimental methods to measure the effect and qualitative methods to understand what happened. A range of before-and-after[20] and quasi-experimental designs[21] may dovetail better with the pragmatic nature of educational innovation in the real world, although randomised controlled trials and step-wedge designs may be ideal.

Maintenance

Once training programmes are established and producing graduates who enter the health system, a variety of other educational research questions arise. Stakeholders will want to know if graduates are appropriately trained for their roles in the health system, what they end up doing after graduation and what impact they are having. Surveys may help to gather feedback from graduates once they are working, and to track how their careers evolve.[17,22]

The impact of graduates on the health system is difficult to evaluate, especially when the number of graduates is relatively small. Research that focuses on the environment closest to the new family physicians may provide the best evidence of initial impact. For example, case studies of how individual family physicians affect their facilities and districts, 360-degree evaluations of how others in the system experience family physicians can be collected as a national survey,[23] and observational studies can compare facilities with and without family physicians.[24] Phenomenological and descriptive exploratory qualitative studies can also obtain the lived experiences and perspectives of family physicians, colleagues and managers.[25] Larger scale ecological effects will usually require a critical mass of family physicians in the health system, showing the relationship between the density of family physicians and key clinical outcomes at district level, and will not be possible for several years.[26]

CONCLUSION

Educational research can support the development of family medicine and primary care education in regions and countries by paying attention to the key research questions and appropriate methods at different stages of development. Faculty members should see educational research as a core activity in creating training programmes that are evidence-based, contextualised, high-quality and aligned with national policy goals.

REFERENCES

1. Maeseneer J. Twenty years of Primafamed Network in Africa: looking back at the future. *Afr J Prim Health Care Fam Med* 2017;9(1):1–2. Available from: http://www.scielo.org.za/scielo.php?script=sci_arttext&pid=S2071-29362017000100047 (Accessed 18 April 2020).
2. Crisp LN. Global health capacity and workforce development: turning the world upside down. *Infect Dis Clin North Am* 2011;25(2):359–367. doi:10.1016/j.idc.2011.02.010
3. Prochaska J, DiClemente C. Toward a comprehensive model of change. In: Miller W, Heather N, eds. *Treating Addictive Behaviours: Processes of Change.* Applied Clinical Psychology. New York: Plenum; 1986: 3–27.
4. Mash RJ, De Villiers MR, Moodley K, Nachega JB. Guiding the development of family medicine training in Africa through collaboration with the medical education partnership initiative. *Acad Med.* 2014;89(8 SUPPL.):S73–7. doi:10.1097/ACM.0000000000000328
5. Moosa S, Downing R, Essuman A, Pentz S, Reid S, Mash R. African leaders' views on critical human resource issues for the implementation of family medicine in Africa. *Hum Resour Health* 2014;12(1). doi:10.1186/1478-4491-12-2
6. Flinkenflögel M, Setlhare V, Cubaka V, Makasa M, Guyse A, De Maeseneer J. A scoping review on family medicine in sub-Saharan Africa: practice, positioning and impact in African health care systems. *Hum Resour Health* 2020;18:1–18. Available from: https://link.springer.com/content/pdf/10.1186/s12960-020-0455-4.pdf (Accessed 18 April 2020).

7. Sururu C, Mash R. The views of key stakeholders in Zimbabwe on the introduction of postgraduate family medicine training: a qualitative study. *Afr J Prim Health Care Fam Med* 2017;9(1). doi:10.4102/phcfm.v9i1.1469

8. Ogundipe RM, Mash R. Development of Family Medicine training in Botswana: views of key stakeholders in Ngamiland. *Afr J Prim Health care Fam Med* 2015;7(1).

9. Mash R, Downing R, Moosa S, De Maeseneer J. Exploring the key principles of Family Medicine in sub-Saharan Africa: international Delphi consensus process. *S Afr Fam Pract* 2008;50(3):60–65. doi:10.1080/20786204.2008.10873720

10. Mash RB, Reid S. Statement of consensus on Family Medicine in Africa. *Afr J Prim Health Care Fam Med* 2010;2(1):4.

11. Couper I, Mash B, Smith S, Schweitzer B. Outcomes for family medicine postgraduate training in South Africa. *S Afr Fam Pract* 2012;54(6).

12. Mash B, Couper I, Hugo J. Building consensus on clinical procedural skills for South African family medicine training using the Delphi technique. *S Afr Fam Pract* 2006;48(10).

13. Akoojee Y, Mash R. Reaching national consensus on the core clinical skill outcomes for family medicine postgraduate training programmes in South Africa. *Afr J Prim Health Care Fam Med* 2017;9(1):1353. doi:10.4102/phcfm.v9i1.1353

14. Mash R, Blitz J, Malan Z, Von Pressentin K. Leadership and governance: learning outcomes and competencies required of the family physician in the district health system. *S Afr Fam Pract* 2016;58(6):232–235. doi:10.1080/20786190.2016.1148338

15. de Villiers M, van Schalkwyk S, Blitz J, et al. Decentralised training for medical students: a scoping review. *BMC Med Educ* 2017;17(1):196. doi:10.1186/s12909-017-1050-9

16. Blitz J, De Villiers M, Van Schalkwyk S. Implications for faculty development for emerging clinical teachers at distributed sites: a qualitative interpretivist study. *Rural Remote Health*. 2018;18(2):4482.

17. Mohamed KG, Hunskaar S, Abdelrahman SH, Malik EM. Scaling up family medicine training in Gezira, Sudan – a 2-year in-service master programme using modern information and communication technology: a survey study. *Hum Resour Health*. 2014;12(1):3. doi:10.1186/1478-4491-12-3

18. Jenkins L, Mash B, Derese A. The national portfolio of learning for postgraduate family medicine training in South Africa: experiences of registrars and supervisors in clinical practice. *BMC Med Educ* 2013;13(1):149. doi:10.1186/1472-6920-13-149

19. De Swardt M, Jenkins LS, Von Pressentin KB, Mash R. Implementing and evaluating an e-portfolio for postgraduate family medicine training in the Western Cape, South Africa. *BMC Med Educ* 2019;19(1):251. doi:10.1186/s12909-019-1692-x

20. Mash R, Malan Z, Blitz J, Edwards J. Improving the quality of clinical training in the workplace: implementing formative assessment visits. *S Afr Fam Pract* 2019;61(6): 264–272. doi:10.1080/20786190.2019.1647639

21. Mash R, Pather M, Rhode H, Fairall L. Evaluating the effect of the practical approach to care kit on teaching medical students primary care: quasi-experimental study. *Afr J Prim Health Care Fam Med* 2017;9(1):1602. doi:10.4102/phcfm.v9i1.1602

22. Crowley LE. An evaluation of postgraduate family medicine training at Stellenbosch University : survey of recent graduates. 2018. Available from: http://scholar.sun.ac.za/handle/10019.1/105170. (Accessed 13 March 2020).

23. von Pressentin KB, Mash RJ, Baldwin-Ragaven L, et al. The perceived impact of family physicians on the district health system in South Africa: a cross-sectional survey. *BMC Fam Pract* 2018;19(1):24. doi:10.1186/s12875-018-0710-0

24. von Pressentin KB, Mash RJ, Baldwin-Ragaven L, et al. The influence of family physicians within the South African district health system: a cross-sectional study. *Ann Fam Med* 2018;16(1):28–36. doi:10.1370/afm.2133

25. Von Pressentin K, Mash R, Baldwin-Ragaven L, Botha R, Govender I, Steinberg W. The bird's-eye perspective: how do district health managers experience the impact of family physicians within the South African district health system? A qualitative study. *S Afr Fam Pract* 2018;60(1):13–20. doi:10.1080/20786190.2017.1348047

26. Von Pressentin KB, Mash RJ, Esterhuizen TM. Examining the influence of family physician supply on district health system performance in South Africa: an ecological analysis of key health indicators. *Afr J Prim Health Care Fam Med* 2017;9(1):1298. doi:10.4102/phcfm.v9i1.1298

CHAPTER 31

Intercultural aspects in primary care educational research

Maham Stanyon

THE IMPORTANCE OF CULTURE IN EDUCATIONAL RESEARCH

Intercultural collaborations are a rich source of learning both professionally and personally. Not only does a cultural lens bring valuable new perspectives, but intercultural research is needed to build an evidence base that facilitates the sensitive translation of concepts across cultures.

Internally, competitive fellowships and academic opportunities draw talent from across the globe, resulting in a primary care workforce that reflects the increased diversity of the patient populations served. Such a workforce can energise teams with new ways of thinking, encouraging, understanding and tolerance. However, intercultural interaction will be subject to cultural differences. This chapter aims to provide insights to help you understand where misunderstandings might occur, and strategies to deal with them should they arise.

CULTURAL FRAMEWORKS

Culture shapes our thoughts, beliefs and behaviours in ways we may be unaware of until we encounter those who experience the world differently.[1] However, defining or claiming expertise in culture is fraught with challenges, as culture is neither a homogenous nor static entity.[2] Even amongst those identifying as the same culture, there will be generational, educational and social class differences that influence the effect of culture.[1] There are inherent dangers associated with cultural stereotyping and compared to national preferences, individual tastes may differ.[3,4] However, this must be balanced with an awareness of the bias imposed by interpreting actions against your standards, rather than in the cultural context they were meant. Therefore, frameworks to conceptualise cultural differences are essential.

Many frameworks exist, with most distinguishing cultures based on their handling of power relationships, the conceptualisation of self and conflict management.[5] Hofstede's cultural dimensions is one commonly used framework (Box 31.1), whilst Figure 31.1 shows Meyer's method of mapping cultures across aspects of business culture.[3,4]

Frameworks such as those by Hofstede and Meyer provide a way to express cultural differences objectively within your research. This is of particular importance when writing your ethics application, as it is essential to thoroughly evaluate your methodology for cultural sensitivities and take steps to mitigate any discomfort. Box 31.2 contains a checklist of points to keep in mind when drafting your ethics application and planning your study.

BOX 31.1 HOFSTEDE'S SIX CULTURAL DIMENSIONS

Geert Hofstede found that cultures differ in their approach in six key areas termed 'dimensions'; each one depicts a scale, allowing each culture to be plotted accordingly. The dimensions consist of:

- **Power distance**, relating to how rigidly hierarchy is applied and enforced
- **Uncertainty avoidance**, the level of stress experienced when dealing with the unknown
- **Individualism versus collectivism**, related to how decisions are made
- **Masculinity versus femininity**, how emotional roles are divided within society
- **Long-term versus short-term orientation**, related to the focus of effort and goals
- **Indulgence versus restraint**, related to the control of human desires in enjoying life

(Adapted from: Hofstede, 2011; p8)

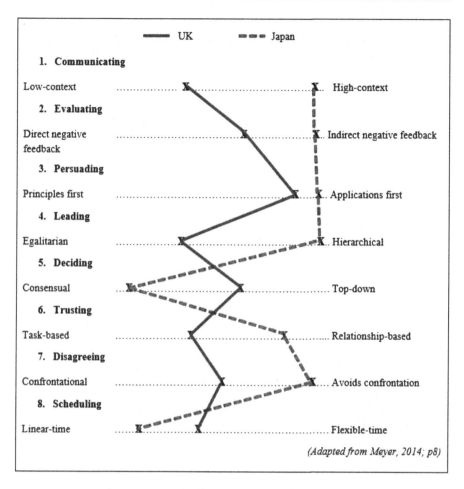

FIGURE 31.1 A 'Culture Map' according to Meyer, depicting the positions of the United Kingdom and Japan across eight aspects of business culture.

SPEECH AND NON-VERBAL BEHAVIOURS

Edward Hall divided cultures into high- and low-context categories based on verbal and non-verbal communication traits (Box 31.3).[6] According to Hall, depending on whether your culture is high- or low-context will determine how you interpret what you hear, and your ideas regarding good communication.[6,7] However, there are limitations to Hall's model, as within all cultures there will be situations requiring both types of communication.[8]

BOX 31.2 CHECKLIST OF CULTURAL ASPECTS WHEN WRITING YOUR ETHICS APPLICATION

- Has an ethics application been written for each participating institution?
- Have sources of funding been checked for international restrictions?
- Is the data shared compliant with the data protection regulations of all participating countries?
- Has the methodology been evaluated for cultural sensitivities?
- Has the welfare of participants been considered from a cultural perspective?
- Do the researchers interpreting the results have suitable cultural expertise to contextualise the results appropriately?
- If participants are being compensated, is the reimbursement culturally appropriate?

BOX 31.3 HALL'S CHARACTERISTICS OF HIGH- AND LOW-CONTEXT CULTURES

HIGH CONTEXT

- Shared understanding/context is required for understanding
- Communication is indirect and nuanced
- Further cues may be obtained through unspoken words
- Truth is flexible to accommodate relationship development
- Verbosity is discouraged
- Communication is relationship-oriented

LOW CONTEXT

- Does not require shared understanding/context for understanding
- Communication is direct and transparent
- Messages are explicitly stated in what is said
- Truth is given priority over relationship building
- Communication is task-orientated

(Adapted from: Cardon, 2008; p401)

High-context communication is opaque and indirect; hearing *how* something is said, or what is *not* said is as important as what is said. To a low-context culture, this seems alien, but to a high-context culture this is normal, and is applied unconsciously to all speech, with the listener decoding these messages along with body language to interpret the meaning.[7] Low-context cultures in contrast value transparent, direct communication, often with messages stated explicitly by those talking to ensure common understanding.[7] When teams contain members from both high- and low-context cultures, adopting a low-context communication approach to ensure everyone understands is recommended.[3]

VIDEO CONFERENCING

Video conferencing poses a challenge due to the loss of non-verbal cues. However, it remains the most efficient and cost-effective method of meeting visually for international projects or for delivering educational interventions across borders. Box 31.4 contains key points to keep in mind for successful video conferencing, particularly when there is a mix of participants from high- and low-context cultures.

The communication traits described earlier still apply when video conferencing, some of which can feel magnified over the video link. This is particularly noticeable when meeting with participants from a culture where

---

BOX 31.4 TOP TIPS FOR SUCCESSFUL VIDEO CONFERENCING

- Be mindful of time zone differences when selecting a time for your meeting
- Take extra care around the first week of March and the first week of November when some countries alter their time zone for daylight saving
- Agree the agenda in advance
- Avoid last-minute changes
- The person speaking should always be visible on screen
- Aim for everyone to join the meeting via video rather than only those offsite appearing by video
- Set ground rules for how people should contribute opinions, e.g. using the raise hand function
- Check with each person if they have anything further to contribute before closing
- Record the meeting and share to allow participants to review aspects they might have missed
- Follow-up the discussion in writing

there is increased use of silence compared to your own. Furthermore, the ability to read and interpret body language is reduced on screen and may mask important signs indicating a person's true meaning.

GIVING FEEDBACK

How feedback is given is culturally constructed, particularly when negative feedback is required. Some cultures welcome direct negative feedback as refreshing and honest, whilst others view direct negative feedback as confrontational and humiliating.[3] The ratio of positive to negative comments within feedback also varies. Some cultures pre-empt a negative comment with one or more positives, whilst at the other extreme are cultures that eschew positive comments unless there has been an exceptional performance.[3]

PRESENTING STYLES

How you construct the narrative of your research and physically interact when delivering your message is influenced by culture. Although medical education research is presented in the background-method-results-discussion-conclusion format, how you explain concepts falls into one of two patterns: an *inductive* or applications-first approach or a *deductive* or principles-first approach. Evidence shows there are cultural preferences for which approach is preferred, which can influence how receptive the audience is to your message.[3]

Additionally, presenter and audience behaviours can be culturally shaped. Hand gestures are mistakenly assumed to be universally understood and can cause offense accidentally.[9,10] Box 31.5 lists some common hand gestures which have negative connotations in some cultures. Other behaviours may also cause surprise if unexpected; for example, in Japan, closing one's eyes during a presentation, a practice known as *inemuri* may be seen, whilst in China, it is acceptable to answer your phone during the presentation.[11]

BOX 31.5   HAND GESTURES TO AVOID DURING INTERNATIONAL PRESENTATIONS

The 'OK' sign – viewed as highly vulgar and offensive in the Middle East, Brazil and Mediterranean countries

Thumbs up – interpreted as an obscene gesture in Iran, Afghanistan and some Mediterranean countries

Raising your hand with the fingers outstretched and palm facing out – a highly offensive insult in Greek culture

(From Archer, 1997 and Sekine, 2015)

SUMMARY

Culture intersects educational research in many ways; from the ethics application, data collection and interpretation to how you present your work. Culture may form part of the research question, bringing exciting developments to the literature, or feature in team interactions promoting a better understanding of your own culture in the process.

Overall, successful intercultural relationships develop over time through mutual hard work and understanding. Refraining from assumptions and getting to know your colleagues as individuals whilst maintaining an awareness of where differences might arise are key to building a successful team culture of your own.

REFERENCES

1. Helman C. *Culture, Health and Illness.* 5th ed. London: Hodder Arnold; 2007.
2. Kumagai AK, Lypson M. Beyond cultural competence: critical consciousness, social justice, and multicultural education. *Acad Med* 2009;84:782–787.
3. Meyer E. *The Culture Map: Decoding How People Think, Lead, and Get Things Done Across Cultures.* International edition. New York: Public Affairs; 2014.
4. Hofstede G. Dimensionalizing cultures: the Hofstede model in context. *Online Readings Psychol Cult* 2011;2(1). https://doi.org/10.9707/2307-0919.1014
5. Inkeles A, Levinson DJ. National character: the study of modal personality and sociocultural systems. In: Linzey G, Aronson E, eds. *The Handbook of Social Psychology IV.* New York: McGraw-Hill; 1969: 418–506.
6. Hall ET. *Beyond Culture.* 1st ed. Garden City, NY: Anchor Press; 1976.
7. Lewis RD. *When Teams Collide: Managing the International Team Successfully.* London: Nicholas Brealey; 2012.
8. Cardon PW. A critique of Hall's contexting model: a meta-analysis of literature on intercultural business and technical communication. *J Bus Tech Comm* 2008;22(4):399–428.
9. Archer D. Unspoken diversity: cultural differences in gestures. *Qual Sociol* 1997;20(1):79–105.
10. Sekine K, Stam G, Yoshioka K, Tellier M, Capirci O. Cross-linguistic views of gesture usage. *Vial-vigo Int J Appl Ling* 2015;12:91–105.
11. Cardon PW, Ying D. Mobile phone use in meetings among Chinese professionals: perspectives on multicommunication and civility. *Glob Adv Bus Comm* 2014;3

CHAPTER 32

Disseminating your primary care educational research

Euan Lawson

INTRODUCTION

Dissemination is an essential part of any research project. No one wants their work to linger unread and unnoticed. The classic dissemination process is well worn: first, complete the research; perhaps submit an abstract and a poster to a suitable conference; then write an academic paper and submit it to journal. That's it. Many people still think that way, perhaps with the addition of a few tweets tagged on the end as a nod to modern social medial channels.

This does still work, but there is a considerable quantity of work that goes into any research, and there are many waypoints where it is possible to engage with the community in a scholarly way. It is worth pausing to think about your aims with dissemination. This might seem self-evident, but it usually bears some reflection. Here are some questions to consider:

- Could your work have a large impact on how people deliver medical education or is it more of an incremental addition to the body of knowledge?
- Will publishing your work in a particular academic journal mean the right people read it?
- How could your work change policy and practice? And where do these people meet, what do they read and how do they come to their decisions? How could you get to them?

- How does this research matter to your career?
- What do other members of the research team want?
- What do your funders (if you have any) expect from you?
- Does your institution have fixed ideas about how your work should be disseminated and the impact your work has?

It should also be pointed out that there are no right answers to these questions. There is not a single correct method to disseminate research, and context is critical. Unpicking that, and if necessary, agreeing the aims with immediate colleagues, institutions and wider stakeholders, is all part of the process.

REFINING THE KEY MESSAGES

Establishing the key messages of your research is an essential element in the process of disseminating your work. It can be painful to squeeze months, sometimes years, of work into a few lines, but you should be able to state them with confidence and clarity.

This refined summary can be used in many different formats. In any article you will know exactly what you need to write to best present your work, in a podcast or interview you can quickly give an accurate précis, and you will know the top line message for your poster. You will be able to compose tweets or Facebook posts, make pertinent comments at conferences, tell colleagues during coffee breaks or meeting at the water cooler and speak with clarity in meetings. It will also help you write your journal article to ensure long-term dissemination of your article in two important but neglected areas: the title and the abstract.

THE TITLE

You should spend time on this. Most people now find papers by combing the internet through search engines and indexes such as PubMed, the journal's own pages, or Google Scholar. This means that titles should be easily understood, with important keywords included. Qualitative studies can be particularly guilty of this, and while the quotes used are often beautifully evocative, there is a very real danger that the paper then skulks in obscurity. The title is your hook to get the reader.

THE ABSTRACT

As a journal editor, it is all too clear that the abstract is often treated as an afterthought. It is dashed off at the end when everyone is in a rush to make the submission. Yet, it will be the single most read section of your paper. We all know this, as we have screened countless hundreds of papers based on the abstract. There are just 150–250 words to inform (and persuade if needed) the reader that your paper has exactly what they need. Spend time on it. Refine it. Write several drafts and get someone else, unfamiliar with your research, to read it and comment. Can they understand what you did and what you found? It is that important. It will drive search engine and directory traffic for years to come.

SOME TIPS ON INTERACTING WITH JOURNALS AND GETTING PUBLISHED

Most research will be written up as a paper and submitted to a journal. Here are some suggestions to help improve those interactions.

- You need to do some market research. Journal selection is essential and there are many options across the spectrum. You may consider open-access journals like *BMC Medical Education* but, unless you are submitting from a country included in the Hinari Access to Research for Health programme, you will need to be able to pay article processing charges. This can be a significant barrier for the under-funded discipline of medical education. There are also several hybrid journals like *Academic Medicine* and *Medical Education* where no costs will be incurred, but only a selection of articles are accepted. By all means, consider reputation, but also consider each journal's core readership and whether it matches your aims for dissemination.
- Do not discount other more specialist publications – if your project had a specific clinical focus, then the speciality journals could be an option. Again, study what they publish and, if unsure, email the editor and ask.
- Read closely the guidance for authors on their websites. Tailor your article according to the journal's requirements. All too often, authors write their paper and then look for a journal. Take a leaf from the book of professional writers, journalists and freelancers. Know the publication and fashion accordingly.
- Write a covering letter but keep it brief and do not oversell the work – your well-crafted title and abstract can do the heavy lifting. Use the name of the editor. It shows you have spent at least a few minutes checking the journal's pages and you are not simply recycling your submission.
- Try not to take it personally if they reject your paper and work to build relationships with editors.

SOCIAL NETWORKS, SOCIAL MEDIA AND BEYOND

Any consideration of dissemination of research these days would not be complete without touching on the subject of social media. However, I would encourage you to broaden your thinking and consider the use of social media as an adjunct to the wider topic of social networking.

THE REAL SOCIAL NETWORK

This may seem terribly old-fashioned, even quaint, but face-to-face contact is not to be under-estimated as a long-term strategy for research dissemination. It is too easy for introverted bookish types to hide behind modern communication platforms that mean we do not have to engage people in actual conversation. Speaking to other people is the highest fidelity way to engage and disseminate.

So, after getting that poster accepted, do not just add it to your CV, and then ignore. Set up your poster at the conference and stand beside it. Talk to people and tell them about your work. Leave a mobile number and tell them to text if they want to ask you questions. Engage with your peers.

Most primary care medical education communities are relatively tight groupings. However, they are not all, usually, conveniently placed in a single workplace. Yet, at conferences, that is exactly what happens. It can be tiring, especially if you are introverted, but that kind of social networking can build long-term relationships that trump the most ardent of tweeters.

Do not ignore the immediate social networks you already have and have cultivated. Send your paper to colleagues in your department and in your faculty. Or send it to colleagues who may be working in similar posts in other institutions. Identify the communities of people who are involved in medical education for primary care. Reach out to them and share.

TWITTER AND OTHER SOCIAL MEDIA

All of the social networking discussed above can also happen online and there is ample opportunity to build networks with people from all over your country and all over the world. That is perhaps the greatest benefit. The real-world impact of Twitter is difficult to quantify and surprisingly limited. It is important to understand how social media contributes to scientific debate, but the link between social media use and citations remains unclear.[1,2]

Developing a social media profile is a long game. It takes many months, if not years, of engagement to make any headway. While rare exceptions exist, the people in the academic community who are social media influencers were already influencers. For individuals, the time and effort of social media needed is an enormous investment that carries opportunity costs. Beware the dopamine hit of social media – mobile phones utilise the same intermittent positive reinforcement that makes gambling machines highly addictive.

DISSEMINATION BEYOND THE USUAL PATH

At this point, you should refer back to your aims for dissemination and use your imagination. The options are numerous: set up a webpage of your own or an institutional microsite; ensure your institutional pages are up to date; create a short video and get your institutional account to feature it; record a podcasting; write opinion articles and letters to the trade press as well as journals. There are few limits here.

It remains the case that publishing articles in academic journals is the central plank of most dissemination strategies, yet it is possible to finesse, even innovate, with a little thought and planning. Start early, consider a range of options beyond the usual pathways and have a clear aim from the outset.

REFERENCES

1. Studenic P, Ospelt C. Do you tweet? Trailing the connection between Altmetric and research impact! *RMD Open* 2020;6:e001034.
2. Tonia T, Van Oyen H, Berger A, Schindler C, Künzli N. If I tweet will you cite? The effect of social media exposure of articles on downloads and citations. *Int J Public Health* 2016;61:513–520.

CHAPTER 33

Future challenges in primary care educational research

Val Wass and Simon Gay

ALIGNING EDUCATION WITH HEALTH CARE DELIVERY

This book reaches fruition at a most pertinent time. As we come to grips with the COVID-19 pandemic, health care delivery will inevitably change. There has been a rapid acceleration to more remote clinical delivery. Education has reacted remarkably swiftly to place learning online.[1] With more virtual consultations, learning through in-person interactions may reduce and move to other interprofessional team members supported by artificial intelligence and robotics. Future health care professionals will deal with higher levels of complexity, weighing probability and risk in new ways, whilst climate change and escalating migration impact on individuals and communities. The World Organization of Family Doctors' (WONCA) commitment for primary care to meet the Sustainable Development Goals[2] will depend on how well training across the continuum of medical education adjusts to meet changing health care demands.

PROVIDING AN EVIDENCE BASE FOR EDUCATIONAL CHANGE

Never has it been more important to critically look, using robust research methodology and judicious application of theoretical frameworks, at how we deliver primary care education. Authentic defensible evidence is essential to substantiate how best to adjust curricular learning outcomes to optimise the opportunities community-based learning offers (Chapter 5). Relying on past methods and anecdote will not work. The theoretical underpinnings of education research (Chapter 2) become of paramount importance as does the need to collaborate with other specialities, especially the behavioural sciences (Chapter 3). Ever increasing global migration of both patients and clinicians places growing pressure on values-based education. The huge deficit in health care workers[3] has to be addressed. Research is essential to understand how to move from traditional hierarchical structures to interprofessional learning (Chapter 8), where doctors may need to follow, not lead, in multi-professional teams. Understanding frameworks for addressing cultural awareness and diversity is of paramount importance (Chapter 31). Stronger participatory design of research projects (Chapter 4) becomes increasingly essential for future research.

THE IMPORTANCE OF DIFFERENTIATING EVALUATION FROM RESEARCH

A crescively important issue is distinguishing evaluation from research. Evaluation has to improve if we are to understand how to respond to COVID-19.[1] Frameworks for evaluation are essential, and must be better built into process (Chapter 27). Studies of educational interventions focussing only on student reaction (i.e. Kirkpatrick level 1[4]) fail to produce the generalisable knowledge needed to inform stakeholders and disseminate findings widely.[5] The challenge is to establish not only what stakeholders learn and how behaviour can be changed, but also to identify how educational interventions impact on patient outcomes. It then becomes crucial to distinguish between research and evaluation. The former shares many attributes with evaluation but, if the aim is to create new knowledge for publication beyond the local community (Chapter 27), careful advance consideration must be given to ethical approval. Ensuring stakeholder consent and protecting confidentiality and anonymity becomes vital (Chapter 13). Failure to do so prevents publication; a pitfall to be avoided if research into the impact of educational interventions is to achieve acceptable validity and reliability (Chapter14) and dissemination (Chapter 31).

RE-IMAGINING MEDICAL EDUCATION TO ADDRESS FUTURE SKILL CHANGE

Aligning education with health care change opens new educational territory. COVID-19 may well have a permanent effect on in-person contact. This arguably must be preserved.[6] As health care becomes progressively community-based, primary care is the obvious context for experiential, transformational learning. Yet research on how trainees learn in this context and when and how it should be delivered is scarce. Mixed methods research with careful design can really impact (Chapter 25). Learning differential diagnosis through hypothetico-deductive reasoning and automatic pattern recognition may be threatened as artificial intelligence takes hold. Handling uncertainty, risk and resilience are critical future attributes. Can they be learnt? It is important to systematically explore what is already known in the wider non-clinical education arena (Chapter 10) before developing well-defined answerable research questions (Chapter 11). A wide range of approaches: Delphi techniques, action research, case base studies, focus groups, content analysis and ethnography (Chapters 18, 20–24, respectively) offer opportunities for mixed methodologies to explore little known areas. Introducing new theoretical frameworks drawn from other disciplines, such as threshold concepts,[7] illustrates how matching methodology to carefully focussed research questions (Chapter 12) could establish the framework's efficacy in helping learners accept uncertainty.

UNDERSTANDING HOW LEARNING IS CONTEXTUALISED ACROSS HEALTH CARE ENVIRONMENTS

Changing health care impacts on learning environments. Systems and processes vary widely across geography, demography and economy. Sadly, we have been slow to learn from resource-poor lower- and middle-income countries,[8] and need to open our eyes to such opportunities. The success of future education research depends on interprofessional collaboration (Chapter 8) developing a critical mass across countries and regions (Chapter 29). It would be a mistake to confine studies to primary care. Integration at the primary-secondary care interface (Chapter 7) is vital. Exploring how students learn from following patients through health care systems, and how different models for longitudinal integrated clerkships impact,[9] is important. Quantitative study design (Chapter 15) and big data collected nationally to map demographic data, academic performance and career choice (Chapter 16) is as yet limited but has great potential. At institutional level, qualitative methodology (Chapter 9) is gaining increasing credibility in understanding the learning environment. The hidden curriculum (Chapter 28) is proving a rich area for revealing dynamic undercurrents impacting, often unintentionally, on learning and career choice.[10] Increasingly, technological advances and social media (Chapter 17) will enhance our ability to explore further.

CONCLUSION

Primary care educational research has never been more crucial if we are to establish the appropriately balanced workforce to meet changing health delivery and the overwhelming health care worker deficit.[3] Raising the profile of academic primary care to learners is key to attracting the brightest and best students into a career in family medicine.[11] Established primary care researchers offer, through this WONCA book, both the theory and tools to underpin this alongside a platform for peer mentoring (Chapter 29). COVID-19 has catalysed change to bring primary care education to the fore; an opportunity we cannot afford to miss.

REFERENCES

1. Gordon M, Patricio M, Horne L, et al. Developments in medical education in response to the COVID-19 pandemic: a rapid BEME systematic review. BEME Guide No. 63. *Med Teach* 2020;42:1202–1215.
2. Pettigrew L, Jan De Maeseneer J, Anderson M-I P, Essuman A, Kidd MR, Haines A. Primary health care and the Sustainable Development Goals. *Lancet* 2015;386:2119–2121.
3. World Health Organisation. No health without a workforce. Available from: https://www.who.int/workforcealliance/knowledge/resources/hrhreport2013/en/ (Accessed 21 November 2020).
4. Kirkpatrick D. Evaluation of training. In: Craig RL, Bittel LR, eds. *Training and Development Handbook*. McGraw-Hill: New York, USA. 1967: 87–112.
5. Sandars J, Brown J, Walsh K. Producing useful evaluations in medical education. *Educ Prim Care* 2017;28:137–140.
6. Dornan T, Gillespie H, Amour D, Reid H, Bennett D. Medical students need experience not just competence. *BMJ* 2020;371:m4298. doi:10.1136/bmj.m4298
7. Neve H. Learning to become a primary care professional: insights from threshold concept theory. *Educ Prim Care* 2019;30:5–8.
8. Crisp N. *Turning the World Upside Down. The Search for Global Health in the 21st Century*. London: Royal Society of Medicine Press Ltd; 2010.
9. Worley P, Couper I, Strasser R, et al. A typology of longitudinal integrated clerkships. *Med Educ* 2016;50:922–932.
10. Royal College of General Practitioners UK. Destination GP: Medical students' experiences and perceptions of general practice. Available from: https://www.rcgp.org.uk/-/media/Files/Policy/A-Z-policy/2017/RCGP-destination-GP-nov-2017.ashx?la=en (Accessed 22 November 2020).
11. Wass V, Petty-Saphon K, Gregory S. By choice not by chance: supporting students towards careers in General Practice. Report for Health Education England and UK Medical School Council 2016. Available from: https://www.hee.nhs.uk/sites/default/files/documents/By%20choice%20-%20not%20by%20chance%20PDF.pdf (Accessed 22 November 20).

CHAPTER 34

Conclusive remarks

Felicity Goodyear-Smith

The aim of this book is to inspire those involved in teaching and training in primary care to research and evaluate their educational endeavours. It caters for those working in both undergraduate and postgraduate settings around the world, and is particularly targeted at the emerging researcher.

We hope this book will help equip you with the skills and tools to actively engage in researching the various components of your programmes, from curriculum development to mode of delivery, especially online in our increasingly virtual world, forms of assessment through to full evaluation of your programmes. Increasingly, big data can enable tracking of our graduates and an understanding of their subsequent contribution to the primary care workforce.

Primary care is increasingly a team activity, and working with others, especially interprofessionally, on designing and conducting your research will provide social connection, support and cross-fertilisation of ideas. Including senior researchers as members of your team will help upskill everyone, as well as support their academic careers by co-authorship of peer-reviewed publications.

Our discipline is eclectic, and so too are the various approaches and methods that can be used in primary care educational research. You can draw from many other disciplines and paradigms, and adapt frameworks and implementation models to research your teaching and learning innovations in the context of your own practice. Your setting may range from the classroom to clinical attachments in a wide range of urban and rural sites globally, as well as a totally virtual environment.

We hope this book provides you with a guide to embarking on primary care educational research. You may also find more comprehensive details of specific primary care research methodologies in our companion book,

How To Do Primary Care Research.[1] Enjoy the process, be proud that you are looking critically at and adding to our evidence base to optimise education, while at the same time enhancing your own academic career.

REFERENCE

1. Goodyear-Smith F, Mash B. *How To Do Primary Care Research.* London, UK: CRC Press; 2018.

Index

Note: Locators in *italics* represent figures and **bold** indicate tables in the text.

Printed in the United States
by Baker & Taylor Publisher Services